Making Sense of Data and Statistics in Psychology

Brian Greer and Gerry Mulhern

palgrave

First published 2002 by
PALGRAVE
Houndmills, Basingstoke, Hampshire RG21 6XS and
175 Fifth Avenue, New York, N.Y. 10010
Companies and representatives throughout the world

PALGRAVE is the new global academic imprint of
St. Martin's Press LLC Scholarly and Reference Division and
Palgrave Publishers Ltd (formerly Macmillan Press Ltd).

ISBN 0–333–62968–X hardback
ISBN 0–333–62969–8 paperback

This book is printed on paper suitable for recycling and made from fully managed and sustained forest sources.

A catalogue record for this book is available from the British Library.

Library of Congress Cataloging-in-Publication Data

Greer, Brian, 1944–
    Making sence of data and statistics in psychology / Brian Greer and Gerry Mulhern.
        p.   cm
    Includes bibliographical references and index.
    ISBN 0–333–62968–X (cloth : alk. paper)
    1. Psychometrics. 2. Psychology – Research – Methodology. I. Mulhern, Gerry. II. Title.
    BF39 .G727 2001
    150'.1'5195 – dc21   2001053261

10   9   8   7   6   5   4   3   2
11 10 09 08 07 06 05 04 03

Printed in China

MAKING SENSE OF DATA AND STATISTICS IN PSYCHOLOGY

Contents

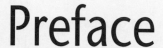

Preface

This book was prompted by our perceived need for a textbook that would present the essentials of statistics and research methods in the style in which we wished to teach our own students.

Our philosophy has developed over the twenty-three years that we have known each other, and the ten years that we worked together. During that time, there have been significant changes to undergraduate and college psychology. Most notable has been the explosion in the number of students wishing to study psychology, resulting in large class sizes and students with diverse backgrounds sitting side-by-side in lectures. Some students will have studied mathematics and statistics to a relatively advanced level, while many more will have a more modest background. Some will relish the prospect of learning about the quantitative aspects of psychology, while others will harbour reservations. This is a reality for groups of psychology students the world over.

A further challenge resulting from larger class sizes has been the increased anonymity of students and the greater sense of 'distance' between teacher and pupil. Students may seldom have an opportunity to discuss ideas or problems with their lecturers, certainly compared to 'our day', and lecturers may not easily be able to identify students who may be experiencing difficulties. This too is a reality in most university and college psychology departments.

A third change has been the staggering increase in the availability and power of computer-based technology within psychology departments. Not very long ago, students and researchers who wanted to analyse their data had to slog away with pencil, paper and a rudimentary calculator. Year by year, technology has become more powerful and affordable. Today, liberal access to powerful computers and statistical packages capable of analysing large data sets at the click of a mouse button is a reality for the vast majority of psychology students. Why do we see this as a challenge? Simply because students have largely lost direct contact with their data, entrusting to computers the tedium of summarising and analysing their numbers.

Moreover, as many have found to their cost, if instructed to do so, computers will 'happily' carry out an incorrect analysis and produce an authoritative printout of garbage. It is important to remember that the ultimate responsibility to make sense of the data lies with the student. This involves interpreting the output of a statistical package and, crucially, having the wherewithal to spot dubious or confusing results.

How, we asked ourselves, could we cater for the needs of students in this changing and challenging climate? How could we present material to large and highly diverse groups of students in a way that all would find relevant? How could we help militate against the greater perceived anonymity of students and pupil–teacher distance? How could we present material so that students might make sense of data and statistical analysis, as well as being able to judge the plausibility of results produced by computers? You the reader can decide the extent to which this book has succeeded in achieving these aims.

NOTE TO TEACHERS

The text has a number of noteworthy features. Throughout, we have placed a strong emphasis on pedagogy, most notably through the use of 'Socratic' dialogues and *'before reading on . . .'* exercises. We hope you find these a positive addition and that you encourage your students to engage with them. You will also notice that the book is highly visual, with some two hundred and fifty figures and tables – this is perhaps its most distinctive feature, reflecting a pedagogic approach that we have found effective with our own large, heterogeneous groups of psychology students.

We have strived to ensure that the dialogues have been presented in a natural, informal style and we have taken great care to identify and ventilate the conceptual challenges that the reader is likely to face – many are based on actual conversations with our own students.

The *'before reading on . . .'* exercises are also based directly on our experience of teaching undergraduates. Typically, these are the short tasks with which we have punctuated our own lectures and tutorials over the years. We would urge you to make use of them in your own teaching and to ensure that students engage with the tasks where they appear in the text, rather than coming back to them later or skipping over them altogether.

A further important feature is the way in which we have grouped statistical tests within chapters. With few exceptions, authors of statistics texts in psychology have tended to deal with parametric and non-parametric methods separately. We see little justification for this approach, since the separation is based, not on what statistical tests *do*, but on whether or not certain assumptions can be made about the data being analysed.

We consider it more pedagogically sound to group the various statistical tests on the basis of their function. Hence, you will see that, following three introductory chapters, most of the rest of the book divides into two strands, based on the two main functions of statistical tests – *comparing* data sets, and *relating* data sets.

A further important feature of the book is that, in each strand, chapters are organised so that concepts introduced at an earlier stage are later revisited and elaborated. Using this approach, examples are first presented descriptively and graphically, while later chapters present a more advanced statistical treatment of these examples.

Thus, in the *comparing* strand, Chapter 4 introduces key concepts relating to the description and graphical display of comparisons between two data sets. These ideas are an extension of those presented in Chapter 3, which deals with the description of single variables. In turn, Chapter 7 shows how these concepts and examples can be extended to formal statistical tests of comparisons between two data sets. In Part 2 of the book, the ideas are extended further to include comparisons of more than two data sets, first descriptively (Chapters 10 and 12), then in terms of statistical tests (Chapters 11 and 13).

In the *relating* strand, Chapter 5 also builds on ideas from Chapter 3 by discussing methods for displaying and describing relationships between two variables. Chapter 8 extends the concepts to formal statistical tests of correlation between two variables, and these are further elaborated in Chapter 14 to include correlation and regression analysis in a multivariate context.

Chapters 6, 9 and 15 straddle both strands. In Chapter 6, the relationship between probability and statistical testing is introduced, which is a necessary preparation for moving from the descriptive statistics in Chapters 4 and 5 to statistical testing in Chapters 7, 8 and beyond.

Chapter 9 is a somewhat pivotal chapter, in which ideas are revisited, drawn together and elaborated. Here key concepts in experimental design, such as control, causation, and validity of experiments, are discussed. The inextricable link between specific research designs and choice of statistical test is also discussed, as is the logic of statistical inference. Chapter 15 concludes matters by drawing together the key themes of the book, including variability, statistical inference and a discussion of some of the controversies surrounding the null hypothesis testing approach to significance testing.

BRIAN GREER
GERRY MULHERN

Acknowledgements

We are particularly grateful to Frances Arnold of Palgrave, who commissioned the book, for her support and infinite patience. She must have wondered at times whether she would ever see the finished product! Thanks also to Philippa English, and to her predecessor, Houri Alavi, for looking after the day-to-day production details with such efficiency and good humour. To Swapna and Maire, love and thanks for your forbearance over several years of gestation and labour. We are also indebted to the many people, too numerous to mention, who had an influence on the final product. James Nicholson, Liz Sproule and Judith Wylie deserve special mention for reading and commenting on the manuscript. Finally, our thanks to the three anonymous reviewers for their constructive and insightful comments which undoubtedly enhanced the final product. Any errors or omissions that remain are ours and ours alone.

BRIAN GREER
GERRY MULHERN

Statistics in psychology

IN THIS
CHAPTER

. . .

. . . we describe our approach to the book and our aims and expectations for its readers. The status of psychology as a science is examined, and the importance of statistical methods within psychology discussed. The nature of variability in psychological research data is also examined, and four main sources of variation identified.

WHAT DOES THIS BOOK OFFER?

This textbook is intended to achieve something that many of its predecessors promised, but too often failed to deliver; that is, to present a clear, concise, non-technical explanation of statistical and methodological concepts in psychology at introductory level (Part 1), and similarly to explore key concepts at post-introductory level (Part 2).

As the title suggests, our approach is to enable you to acquire a 'feel' for data, as well as a pragmatic competence in statistical techniques. We aim to provide a conceptual framework that allows you to get the most from your data. Since, nowadays, students seldom, if ever, need to compute statistics by hand, we stress an understanding of principles and concepts, rather than procedural or technical understanding. Throughout the book, we place considerable emphasis on principles of **exploratory data analysis** (EDA) and on encouraging you to acquire fluency in the use of visual representations.

Since we are psychologists, our focus is more on data analysis than statistical theory, so, on occasion, we have chosen to simplify concepts in a way that a 'hard' statistician might wish to elaborate or qualify. We make no apology for this.

OUR PHILOSOPHY AND APPROACH

In writing this book we have attempted to strike an appropriate balance between the curricular imperatives of psychological statistics and the need to acknowledge the realities of life as a psychology student coming to terms with statistics, probably for the first time.

We recognise that the majority of students using this text will be members of large classes, learning statistics in the relatively impersonal setting of lectures and large laboratory classes. Many students, rightly or wrongly, find large classes intimidating and unconducive to asking questions. A consequent risk of students' failure to clarify important concepts as the need arises may be slow progress, reduced momentum and, in some cases, disenfranchisement. This is a reality.

We are also conscious that, in general, groups of psychology students tend to be heterogeneous in terms of ability, motivation and academic background. While, for some, psychology may be their main academic interest, others will be taking it as a minor or subsidiary subject. Moreover, some students will have studied science and mathematics to an advanced level, while many more will have taken humanities and social sciences. A substantial proportion of the latter will, to a greater or lesser extent, find the idea of learning statistics daunting, if not aversive. This too is a reality.

Our aim in writing this book is to present statistical concepts in a way that will engage all students, irrespective of ability, academic background, or attitude to learning statistics. In doing so:

- we have kept the written text relatively short and to the point, liberally peppering it with figures and illustrations;

- in order to help orientate the reader, new concepts and terms are printed in **bold** type;

- where possible, we have avoided technical jargon, mathematical symbols and formulae – many other textbooks state this aim but merely pay lip-service to it;

- we have gone even further by limiting the arcane terminology of psychological statistics, such as 'central tendency', which is an unnecessary legacy of the past;

- in order to avoid 'getting in the way' of the statistical concepts under consideration, we use vivid, simple examples;

- similarly, we use real data sets for authenticity, as well as smaller bespoke, though plausible, sets designed to make a specific point. On occasion, we juxtapose two alternative or contrasting data sets in order to emphasise a particular concept;

- through the use of dialogues, we discuss, in everyday language, the sorts of questions that typically occur to students;

- active learning is encouraged through regular use of *'Before reading on . . .'* activities sandwiched within the text;

■ from our experience gained over many years, we try to anticipate and pre-empt the conceptual difficulties that students may encounter; and

■ we assume that all students will have ready access to one of the popular computer-based statistical packages, although we have not geared the book to any one in particular.

Figure 1.1 presents a schematic guide to chapters. You will see that, following this introductory chapter, the rest of the book divides largely into two strands, based

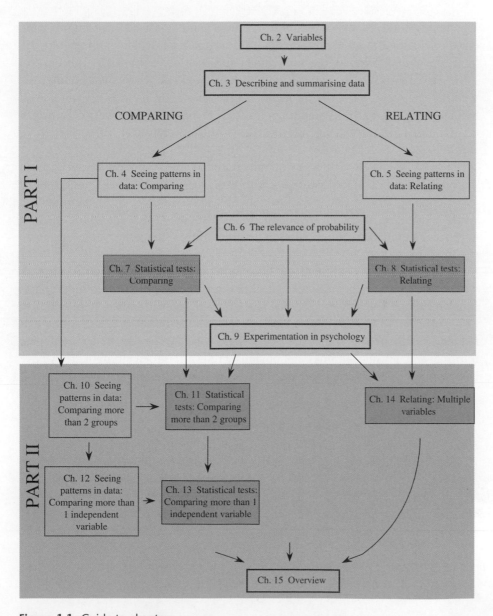

Figure 1.1 Guide to chapters

on the two main functions of statistical tests – *comparing* data sets, and *relating* data sets (more of this later). An important feature of the book is that, in each of these two strands, chapters are organised so that ideas introduced at an earlier stage are later revisited and elaborated. We hope you will find this approach to learning effective, as you are encouraged to progress gradually with an opportunity to revise and build upon earlier material.

HOW TO USE THIS BOOK

This text is not a 'cookbook' or an instruction manual. Those intending to whip out a calculator and set about finding out *how to do* a particular statistical test will be disappointed. Such is the ubiquity of information technology, the days of having to carry out your own calculations have well and truly gone. In any case, we take the view that working through calculations by hand is overrated as a means of gaining an understanding of a test. Recognising this, we focus instead on the rationale underlying statistical tests and on statistical interpretation of results.

The book has been written as an integrated whole, with the sequencing of material carefully planned. Students with little statistical knowledge and limited experience of data handling are strongly advised to start at the beginning and work though to the end. Experienced readers may prefer a more flexible approach, although we would advise that they too should adhere more or less to the intended sequence.

As has already been indicated, we have punctuated the text at regular intervals with *Before reading on . . .* activities and questions. Please resist the temptation to skip over these. They are an essential part of our pedagogic approach, intended to encourage you to process information actively. Similarly, the *Student/Lecturer* dialogues are an extremely important pedagogic vehicle. The fact that they appear informal and, possibly at times, not obviously relevant is their strength. They have been written carefully for a specific purpose and each contains 'powerful ideas'.

OK, SO WHY STATISTICS?

Student: I became a psychology student because I'm curious about why people behave as they do. I'm not even sure I will want to become a psychologist when I graduate – at the moment, I'm interested in advertising.

Lecturer: That's not unusual; many psychology graduates use their degree as a basis for pursuing a career outside psychology.

Student: I have to say I'm a bit surprised and daunted by the amount of statistics and research methods we're expected to learn. I'm really only interested in the subject matter of psychology, and so are a lot of my friends. I have no interest in statistics, or anything mathematical. Besides, in studying human behaviour; individuals cannot be reduced to mere numbers. So, why are we expected to study statistics?

Lecturer: First let me reassure you that statistics is not some arbitrary hurdle you have to jump over at the whim of a psychology lecturer. Statistics and research methods are among the most valuable subjects you will learn.

Student: Why is that? They don't interest me and, as I said, people can't be reduced to numbers.

Lecturer: Spend a moment or two thinking about some of the psychological facts you have learned on your course so far.

Student: Actually, I've found there aren't too many facts as such. There are lots of theories and ideas, and some major disagreements and controversies.

Lecturer: Why do you think that is?

Student: Well, because researchers have different ideas about the processes underlying behaviour.

Lecturer: And how do they go about forming and developing these ideas?

Student: Usually, they carry out research to test their ideas.

Lecturer: You've basically answered your own question. In a nutshell, the reason why you need to learn about statistics and research methods lies in the fact that psychology is first and foremost an **empirical** discipline. By that I mean that psychological knowledge is acquired through systematic gathering of data, in a variety of forms, and the subsequent analysis and interpretation of these data. Think about some of the major debates in psychology.

Student: What, like nature versus nurture, or different theories of schizophrenia?

Lecturer: What do you notice about the substance of these debates?

Student: Now you mention it, the discussion nearly always focuses on the way the research was carried out, or what the results mean.

Lecturer: True, indeed, much of the debate in psychology consists of critiquing methods and procedures used by researchers to support their own ideas or to counter someone else's. Wouldn't it be more satisfying if you knew something about experimentation and statistics, so that you could do some critiquing of your own?

Student: I suppose so, but two researchers holding incompatible views can't both be right, can they?

Lecturer: It's not so much a question of right and wrong in any absolute sense. As you will see, it has more to do with interpretation. In studying psychology, your task is to evaluate the evidence and come to your own conclusions. Sometimes you will agree with psychologists' interpretations of their findings; at other times you will be less convinced.

Student: But, in order to do that, don't I need to be able to make an informed judgement about the quality of the research and the strength of the data?

Lecturer: Precisely! In order to interpret empirical findings and evaluate the researcher's methods, it is essential that you know statistics and research methods. Incidentally, this expertise will prove useful far beyond the realm of psychology. You need the same powers of critical evaluation and probabilistic reasoning in everyday life, and in virtually every area of employment, including advertising.

Student: Since you put it that way. . . .

Do you recognise yourself in any of the above dialogue? The chances are that you do. Having taught statistics for more than fifty years between the two of us, if we had a pound (or a dollar) for every time one of our students questioned the need to study statistics, we would both be very wealthy!

VARIABILITY IN PSYCHOLOGY

Of course, the fact that psychology is an empirical discipline is a necessary but not sufficient reason for needing to use statistics. Imagine if we lived in a world in which everybody was the same, so that people were identical in every respect, with the same genetic code, physical characteristics, mental capacities, opinions, tastes, ambitions, socioeconomic status, lifestyle, personality, health, life-span, educational qualifications, environmental influences, and so on. Imagine too that all other animals were similarly uniform. Furthermore, suppose we were able to measure or quantify every one of these features with complete precision. In such a world, psychologists would have little need for statistics. Research would merely involve measuring some characteristic or other. What is more, since there would be no variation, measurements of a single person would generalise with complete precision to the entire population. The only statistics that would be required would be the most rudimentary description of these measurements. Even the most basic summary statistics would be redundant.

Hence, it is not the empirical nature of psychology *per se* that gives rise to the need for statistics and research methods; rather, it is the fact that psychology is an empirical discipline in a world of variability, uncertainty and inaccuracy. Given the nature of living things, such variability is inherent in all human, biological and social sciences. Indeed, more generally, the popular view of science as yielding definitive answers has long been untenable, even in the so-called 'pure' or 'natural' sciences, where results are seldom conclusive and frequently contradictory. One only has to think of hotly-debated topics in physics, such as whether the properties of light are best explained by wave or particle theory.

TAMING VARIABILITY

In studying behaviour, psychologists must somehow cope with the variation and uncertainty that is such an essential characteristic of the world in which we live. That is where both **research methods** and **statistics** come in. As you will see later, the two go hand-in-hand. The term 'research methods' refers to a set of procedures and techniques for data collection in situations of variability, while 'statistics' is a set of techniques for exploring, summarising and making sense of the data collected. A host of statistical techniques have been designed to cope with variation and uncertainty in data, and each is linked inextricably to the particular research method used to generate the data in the first place. In later chapters, you will see how various statistical techniques are linked to specific research designs.

In statistics, the essential tool for coping with variation and uncertainty that are such essential characteristics is **probability** theory. Chapter 6 describes in some detail how a knowledge of probability helps us to draw conclusions about data.

EVERYDAY STATISTICS

While a term like 'probability' is technical and mathematical, you should bear in mind that we all use ideas of probability regularly in our daily lives. Upon hearing a weather forecast of a 70 per cent chance of rain, you are much more likely to reach for your umbrella than for a forecast of a 5 per cent chance of rain. You would also be surprised to hear that it was likely to snow on Midsummer's Day. You may be familiar with dilemmas faced by investors as to whether to buy shares or to put their money into lower-risk options. In deciding to travel on an aeroplane, or not to eat beef, or to give up smoking, or not to practice safe sex, or to buy a lottery ticket, you are intuitively making probabilistic judgements.

Individuals who apparently flout the risks may be considered by others, and perhaps even by themselves, as behaving irrationally. More often, however, it is simply that people have different thresholds for what they consider to be 'acceptable risk', or they may weigh the risk against competing factors.

A possible exception may be the decision to buy a lottery ticket. In the UK, the chance of winning the jackpot is approximately 14 000 000 to 1. Put into context, this means that, if you were to buy a ticket two hours before the draw, you are more likely to be dead by the time the draw is made than you are to have won the jackpot. In spite of these widely publicised odds, millions of people opt for a weekly flutter (including one of the authors of this book, though emphatically not the other – a clear illustration of human variability!).

The important point is that we all appear to make these probabilistic judgements quite naturally. Clearly, the better informed we are about the processes underlying uncertainty, the more likely we are to make sound decisions. In the context of psychological research, statistics provides a formal framework to enable you to make similar judgements about data.

CAUSES OF VARIABILITY

Among the many sources of variation that afflict psychological research, we can identify four broad clusters:

Measurement variation

Errors in measurement, perhaps the most obvious causes of variability in data, are present in all empirical disciplines. Indeed, variations in astronomical measurements were one of the first contexts within which statistical theory developed. One source of variation is a consequence of the sensitivity, or calibration, of measuring instruments. Put simply, a measurement is only as good as the instrument that produces it. Even for physical characteristics, such as weight or height, instruments have limited sensitivity, and measurements are recorded to the nearest unit of calibration, for example, grams or millimetres.

Variation may also occur due to inaccuracies in measuring instruments. These may be systematic (leading to consistent over- or under-estimation), or they may be random (leading to unsystematic variation from one measurement to the next). The former is likely to prove less problematic than the latter in research, in that systematic measurement errors do not affect the overall pattern of measurements. Indeed, if the magnitude of the error is known, it can be corrected readily by addition to, or subtraction from, the measurement as appropriate.

Situational variation

It may be stating the obvious to suggest that the behaviour of individuals can be affected by environmental conditions, such as time of day, room temperature, appearance of the researcher, or test instructions. Again, these may have a consistent effect on all participants, particularly if the researcher makes an effort to keep situational factors constant. More problematically, conditions may vary randomly from one participant to another, sometimes unavoidably. It may, for example, be a practical necessity to schedule participants throughout the day.

Individual variation

It is self-evident that, on any measure, whether physical or psychological, people display substantial **individual differences**, a term used widely in the psychological literature. Such differences are undoubtedly the most important source of variability in psychological research. Much of the variation is the result of physical and psychological 'traits' which can be considered fixed within, but which differ between, individuals. Many research designs and statistical methods originated from the necessity to cope with individual differences of this sort.

There is, of course, another important cause of individual variation, namely the tendency for individuals to vary in their behaviour or performance from one occasion to the next. For example, if you were to measure a person's reaction time on ten successive occasions, you would find marked differences in performance across the ten sessions. Similarly, you might assess a person's mood on a particular day, only to find it had changed radically the next. This within-individual 'state' variability can arise from natural cycles and rhythms, or from a host of situational factors within a person's everyday life. Of course, since participants are often tested on a one-off basis, performance reflects an individual's state at one, somewhat arbitrary, point in time.

You may find a golfing analogy useful for contrasting between- and within-individual differences. In a tournament, such as the US Masters, competitors play a round of golf on each of four successive days. Between-individual variation is reflected in golfers' scores after each round, and more especially their overall position on the leaderboard at the end of the tournament. Within-individual variation, on the other hand, is indicated by the change in each individual golfer's score across the four days, irrespective of that of other competitors.

Sample variation

As you will see in later chapters, most psychological research involves using data from samples, drawn from a population in order to form general conclusions about the population as a whole. Just as in the case of individual variation, the data from one sample can differ markedly from another because of differences between the individuals making up the samples. Moreover, some samples may give a fair reflection of their parent population, while others may provide a distorted picture. In psychological research, great care must be taken to try to ensure that samples are representative of their populations, so that variability across a number of samples is minimised. Again, as you will see later, various research designs and statistical techniques have been designed to help researchers cope with sampling variation.

IS PSYCHOLOGY A SCIENCE?

In the past, some psychologists have tended to get bogged down with this well-trodden question. Considerable time and energy has been devoted to establishing psychology's scientific credentials. In our view, it is not particularly helpful to think along the lines of the scientific status of psychology. Instead, we consider it more important to focus on the empirical nature of the discipline, guided by the scientific principles of objectivity and rigour. While the collection and analysis of quantitative data play a central role, we should bear in mind that psychology is an eclectic, interdisciplinary subject that relies on a wide range of methodological approaches, including experiments, surveys, case studies, questionnaire studies, test construction, discourse analysis, semi-structured interviews, ethnography, meta-analysis, and computer modelling.

Although these different empirical approaches may appear to have little in common, they all involve the systematic gathering and objective analysis of evidence. As such, each has its role in the 'science of behaviour' and mental life. In this book, we do not attempt to cover the full gamut of empirical approaches to psychological research. Our primary focus is on quantitative methods and analysis, which are by far the most common. In particular, we are concerned with the empirical approach represented in Figure 1.2.

In its basic form, the researcher (i) identifies a topic and specifies the goals of the research; (ii) formulates one or more precise research questions (called **hypotheses**); (iii) devises a study to address these questions (called **research design**); (iv) gathers numerical information about these questions (called **data collection**); (v) summarises and evaluates this information (called **statistical analysis**); and (vi) draws appropriate conclusions (called **interpretation**).

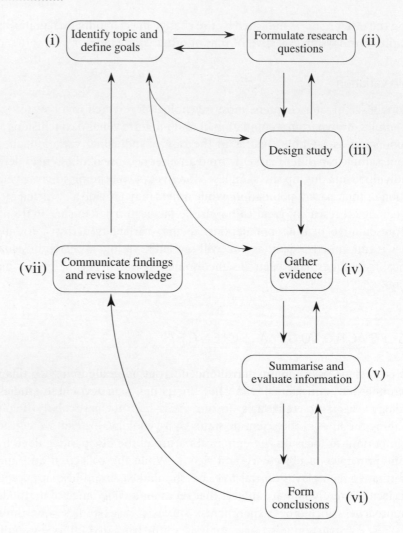

Figure 1.2 The empirical process

Finally, (vii) the results of the study are communicated (called **dissemination**), and integrated with existing knowledge. As the various arrows on the diagram suggest, the process is not necessarily sequential, but may involve iteration and feedback between the various sub-stages. In this book, we focus on the basic cycle in (i)–(vii).

INTERRELATIONSHIP OF THEORY AND EXPERIMENTATION

The iterative processes of feedback and modification, as well as the revision of existing knowledge on the basis of new findings, typify empirical research in psychology and other similar disciplines. Indeed, without this 'experimentation/

theory cycle', psychological research would fail to progress. Instead, we would be left with a collection of fragmented facts. In order that research on any topic can move forward, hypotheses must be rooted in current knowledge of the topic, the data collected must allow the predictions contained in the hypotheses to be tested, and the outcomes must be assimilated into the current body of knowledge, so that the process can begin again.

OBSERVATION VERSUS INTERVENTION

One of the primary goals of science is to provide explanations of what *causes* a particular event or phenomenon to occur. In psychology, the issue of causal explanations of behaviour has long been a hot potato. There is considerable overlap between this debate and arguments regarding the scientific status of psychology, although they are distinct questions.

Two contrasting empirical approaches in psychology may be identified. In the first, researchers undertake experiments, typically laboratory-based and involving active intervention and control of experimental conditions, with relatively small numbers of participants. This approach has become known as the **experimental method**. In the other, researchers observe or measure people's behaviour without direct intervention or control of conditions, typically involving relatively large samples of participants, and often in natural settings. These studies are known as **correlational** or **observational** designs.

Student: I can see there are two basic approaches, but I don't see why the distinction is important.

Lecturer: Actually, as a researcher, it is important to know which method you are using, and that your choice can have important consequences. Let me give you an example. Say you are interested in the effect of sleep deprivation on people's reaction time. How might you use the experimental method to investigate the effect?

Student: You would take a group of people and control the amount of sleep they could have, then measure their reaction times.

Lecturer: Explain how would you do that in a little more detail.

Student: Well, say you had twelve people and you allowed four of them to sleep for two hours before wakening them, another four could be wakened after four hours, and the remaining four after six hours. You would also measure each group's response times when they woke up and look to see if there were differences between the groups.

Lecturer: OK, say you found quite large differences – what would you conclude?

Student: That the amount of sleep affected people's reaction times.

Lecturer: Can you think of any other explanation?

Student: All things being equal, no. That's to say, assuming the three groups were broadly similar in terms of general characteristics, and providing I was sensible and careful about how I treated the people, I think it would its a pretty safe conclusion.

continued

Lecturer: Now, how would you go about investigating the same question using observational methods?

Student: Well, you would just have to find people who had slept for different periods of time and measure their reaction times. I'm not quite sure how you would ensure a spread of sleep deprivation – maybe you could wait outside a local factory and ask people who had just come off the night shift.

Lecturer: So, you're saying that you would end up with a group of people, all of whom had slept for different lengths of time? How, then, would you examine the relationship between sleep deprivation and reaction time?

Student: Basically, by looking to see if, in general, those with less sleep had different response times from those with lots of sleep and those with middling amounts.

Lecturer: Say you found large differences. What could you conclude this time?

Student: Pretty much the same as last time – that the amount of sleep affects reaction time.

BEFORE READING ON . . .

Think about the dialogue so far. Do you agree with the student's conclusions?

. . . now read on

Lecturer: Let's look again at your last conclusion. Might there be other explanations for the differences?

Student: Hmm, I'm not sure.

Lecturer: Well, remember you said that, for the experimental approach, as long as you could assume that the three groups were equivalent in everything except amount of sleep, you could assume that sleep deprivation affected reaction time.

Student: Yes – ah, so you're asking me the same question again. Right, well, since I did not intervene by manipulating the amount of sleep, I just had to take whoever came along.

Lecturer: Can you safely assume that those people with less sleep were otherwise equivalent to those with moderate sleep, and in turn to those with more sleep?

Student: No – for a start, the ones with little sleep might have come from the night shift, or a club, or whatever.

Lecturer: Indeed, or some may be have been rampant insomniacs out looking for a drugstore.

Student: Or werewolves, even!

Lecturer: Hmm! The important thing to remember is that, in the observational study, there may have been some underlying factor, or factors, that influenced both the amount of sleep participants had, and that also determined reaction time. For example, suppose the sleep-deprived individuals tended to be older than their well-slept counterparts.

Student: So, while it might seem that sleep deprivation had influenced reaction time, in reality there is no direct link between the two.

Lecturer: Right – put another way, it might not be a **causal** relationship.

Student: And that's because the study was observational? So the fact that I could infer a causal link in the experiment was because the amount of sleep was carefully manipulated, and this allowed me to assume that any differences between my groups was caused by this intervention?

Lecturer: Correct – assuming you took the necessary precautions to ensure your three groups were equivalent in all other relevant respects.

Student: What precautions are those?

Lecturer: We'll see in Chapter 9.

Student: Incidentally, does that mean that the observational approach is not scientific, but the experimental one is?

Lecturer: That's an interesting question, and there's no simple answer. Certainly, it's true that one approach is called experimental, and the other non-experimental, and some psychologists equate this with the former being scientific and the latter unscientific. Personally, I think this is wrong. I can think of some observational studies that make very good science and some experimental studies that make very bad science. The important thing in all empirical work, whatever the approach, is to strive for rigour and objectivity in the methods used.

CHAPTER REVIEW

Following a discussion of our philosophy and ambitions for the book, we introduced a number of key issues relating to research methods and statistics within psychology. We argued that it is essential to have a sound grasp of statistical concepts in order to understand the empirical aspects of the discipline, as well as a pragmatic sense of how to deal with the ubiquitous influences of variability and uncertainty in psychological data. We also suggested that arguments about the scientific standing of psychology are largely irrelevant and possibly unhelpful.

Making sense of basic designs

Variables 2

IN THIS
CHAPTER
. . .

. . . the methods used to generate the raw material for statistical analysis, namely numerical data, are surveyed. We consider the range of ways in which experimental psychologists go about measuring what they are interested in, and the types of numbers that are produced by these measurement procedures. The key concept of variable as a theoretical entity that can be measured and expressed as a number on a single scale is introduced, and illustrated by typical examples from psychological research. The basic idea of psychological research as the exploration of relationships between variables through data is outlined, with examples.

WAYS OF MEASURING PEOPLE (AND OTHER ANIMALS)

For statistical analysis you need numerical data, and for numerical data you must have ways of measuring what you are interested in. A great deal of effort on the part of scientists in general, and psychologists in particular, goes into devising ways of measuring. Physicists apply great theoretical and technical expertise in measuring the temperatures of distant stars and the properties of sub-atomic particles; psychologists must be equally ingenious in measuring subtle aspects of the behaviour, personality, feelings and the mental life of humans (and other animals).

Here are some examples – intended to be representative rather than to provide an exhaustive survey of all the possibilities – from the measurement repertoire of experimental psychology.

DIRECT PHYSICAL MEASUREMENTS

Historical examples include phrenology (the study of the supposed links between areas of the brain and human propensities through the measurement of parts of the skull) and anthropometry (the study of body measurements). While such approaches have now largely been discredited, they are of great historical interest, and made very important contributions to the development of psychological theory and statistical methods.

In some areas of applied research, such as ergonomics, body measurements like height, weight, grip strength, heart rate and so on are of interest and can be measured using appropriate apparatus. More indirect physiological measures include galvanic skin response (which may give an indication of level of stress, for example) and scans of brain activity (which researchers are beginning to link to mental processes).

OBSERVATIONS

The behaviour of animals, children or adults can be observed in environments varying from **naturalistic** to highly **controlled**, and with or without direct **intervention** by the experimenter. Such observations may be **qualitative** and described in verbal terms (as in a great deal of Piaget's work in cognitive development), or **quantitative**. For example, the frequency of occurrence of a predefined behaviour may be noted, as in counting the number of times a boy or girl playing in a school interacts with 'male' and 'female' toys. Another example would be measuring the amount of time mice placed in the same cage spend fighting with each other.

PERFORMANCE MEASURES

People can be asked to perform any variety of tasks, and aspects of their performance such as speed, accuracy or productivity can be measured. For example, typing skill could be measured by the amount of text typed in a given time, in conjunction with the number of errors made. A rat could be 'asked' to run a maze with a food reward at the end, and its performance measured by the number of wrong turns, and the time taken. Exams might be thought of as a particular, and complex, form of performance measure.

SELF-REPORTS

As long as they have the necessary skills, people can be asked to report things about themselves either verbally or in writing (or some other form of physical recording). A simple example would be a perception experiment in which the participant has to judge whether two stimuli are the same or different on some dimension, and report that judgement to the experimenter. A more complex example would be if the participant is asked, say, 'On a scale of 1 to 10, how anxious are you?'.

A more developed form of this approach is the questionnaire aimed at measuring something in particular. You may be familiar with this sort of exercise in magazines. Under the headline *How sensitive are you to others?* you are asked to answer questions such as:

You are eating out with a number of friends, and one of them asks 'Do you mind if I smoke?'. You do mind.
  Do you say:

(a)   *Yes, it's bad for my health.*

(b)   *No, that's okay.*

(c)   *You should have more concern for others.*

At the end, there is a key that awards points for each answer chosen; you add them up, and are told how, if you scored 46–50 you are too good to be true, and so on. Questionnaires used in psychological research (apart from some technical refinements) are not all that different – see the example below on measuring attitude to computers.

SUBJECTIVE RATINGS

Clearly, some characteristics of people are more difficult to measure than others. In many cases, you can at least ask a panel of people to make subjective judgements, and combine their judgements into a single figure (as is done in ice skating). For example, videotapes of pupils in a classroom could be shown and the panel asked to rate how well each pupil behaved, say on a scale of 1 to 10. Averaging the ratings would give overall measures that could be used in statistical analysis.

NATURE OF DATA GENERATED

Consider a particular number, say 4. If you think about it, we use 4 in many different ways. For a start, we can distinguish between counting and measuring (compare *there are 4 bottles of milk* and *there are 4 pints of milk in the jug*, for example). When a child says 'I am 4 years old', she does not mean exactly 4 (unless it happens to be her birthday), but rather somewhere between 4 and 5 years old. Four can also be used to indicate position in a sequence, as in Henry the Fourth. It can be used for identification purposes (for example, a number 4 bus). And so on . . .

Note that the way in which the number is used determines which arithmetical operations can validly be applied. It makes sense to say that 4 bottles of milk is 1 fewer than 5 bottles of milk, and twice as many as 2 bottles. It makes sense to say that 4°C is 1°C less than 5°C, but it does *not* make sense to say that 4°C is twice as warm as 2°C (think about why not – this will be discussed below). The player in a football team wearing the number 4 shirt is not twice as *anything* as the player wearing the number 2 shirt. You should be able to think of many examples – often they are turned into jokes of a kind as in, 'If Henry the Eighth had six wives, how many did Henry the Fourth have?'.

The most natural use of numbers is for counting discriminable entities (not necessarily physical objects). That's why the positive whole numbers, 1, 2, 3, 4 . . . , are called *natural numbers*. Very often the collection of data in psychological experiments involves counting the number of times something happens – for example, the number of errors a pupil makes on a test, the number of times a rat stands on its hind feet during a given period of time, the number of different uses a person can think of for a barrel (a measure of creativity).

Other numbers represent quantities that can vary continuously and *fill in* the gaps between the natural numbers. An obvious example of something that varies continuously is weight. Intuitively, you can think of weight increasing slowly as you grow, and corresponding to a continuum of numbers associated with some unit of measurement, such as grams. A number line provides a powerful way of forming an image to think about it. For statistical purposes, the numbers between whole numbers can be represented as decimals, to some given level of accuracy. However, data such as weights and heights are often measured to the nearest gram or centimetre.

LEVELS OF MEASUREMENT

The numerical data generated by measuring take many different forms. As will become clear throughout this book, this diversity has crucial implications for the design of experiments and the type of statistical analyses that are appropriate. The various types of number, with differing properties, that are generated by measurement procedures are often referred to by statisticians in terms of four so-called **levels of measurement**, corresponding to measurement scales with increasingly strong properties, as follows:

Nominal scale

This level corresponds to measurement in a minimal sense, in which numbers are used merely as names to distinguish categories, and have none of the properties we would normally associate with numbers (such as relative size). In this case, numbers are used merely as labels for categories into which people may be divided. An example would be nationality. If an experimental investigation of humour was targeting English, French, German and Italian people, then, for convenience, the numerical labels 1, 2, 3, 4 might be attached to people of each of these four nationalities respectively. Any distinguishable symbols could be used just as well, but numerical coding is convenient (and is required for some statistical computer packages). Which numerical label goes with which nationality is arbitrary, and of course there is no sense in which the particular labelling above implies that Italians are higher than Germans on anything, or that Italians are twice as anything as the French.

The simplest case of a nominal measure is when there are only two categories – **dichotomous** data, to use the technical term ('dichotomous' meaning 'cut in two'). An obvious example is gender.

Ordinal scale

Here, the extra ingredient is that the numbers in the scale have a definite order and appropriate inferences can be drawn because of that. By way of example, an investigator looking at the mathematical ability of children in a class might ask the teacher to use subjective judgement to rank the children in this respect. Assuming alphabetical ordering, letters A, B, C . . . could be used just as well (as long as the class didn't have more than 26 members). It is appropriate to conclude that the child ranked 4 (starting from the best) is judged better than the one ranked 5, but not as good as the one ranked 3. However, is not appropriate to conclude that the differences between the children ranked 3 and 4 and those ranked 7 and 8, for example, are the same – it could be that the third best child is *just* better than the fourth, but the seventh is a *lot* better than the eighth. Similarly, it would be nonsensical to conclude that the child ranked 4 is twice as bad (whatever that would mean) as the child ranked 2.

In the example just discussed, there is a single ranking of all the cases, and each rank corresponds to one case. In other situations, each of the ranks may correspond to many cases. For example, suppose the teacher was asked instead to assess each child on mathematical ability as follows: 1 – outstanding; 2 – above average; 3 – average; 4 – below average; 5 – weak. Here again, a rank of 4 is between 3 and 5, but the differences between 3 and 4, and 4 and 5 cannot be assumed equivalent, and in no sense does a rank of 4 represent twice as *anything* as a rank of 2.

Assigning numbers to ranks facilitates the calculation of various statistics and the coding of data for computer analysis.

Interval scale

Measurement on an interval scale implies all the properties of an ordinal scale, but in addition it has the property that differences, or intervals, may be considered equal. An example is temperature, as measured in degrees Centigrade, say. The difference between 8°C and 12°C is equivalent to that between 33°C and 37°C. It would take the same amount of heat energy to raise the temperature of a fixed amount of water by 4°C in both cases. However, it does not make sense to say that 8°C is twice as warm as 4°C, since Centigrade is not measured on a scale with an absolute zero; rather, zero on this scale is the temperature at which water freezes.

Ratio scale

Finally, on a ratio scale, it makes sense to compare two numbers on the scale in terms of their ratio, because zero on such a scale really means 'nothing' of what is being measured. Weight is a clear example – zero is the weight of nothing, the reading on a balance when there is nothing on it. As a consequence, the ratio of two measures is meaningful – a baby mouse of 40 grams is twice as heavy as one of 20 grams (two of the lighter mice would balance one of the heavier on a balance, for example).

DERIVED VALUES

Many numbers that become the grist for statistical mills are not simple direct measurements as such, but rather the results of more or less complex procedures. For example, consider an experiment in which reaction time is being measured (that is, the time it takes someone to react to a stimulus – for example, by pressing a button when a light comes on). It would be possible simply to measure the time that this takes (for example, by using apparatus interfaced with a computer that can determine when the light went on and when the button was pressed, and working out the time interval between these events). The disadvantage is that you would be relying on a single measurement of a capability that is subject to considerable fluctuation, as can be demonstrated by asking someone to carry out this task repeatedly. Accordingly, it is much better to make the measurement several times and take some sort of average of the results. This average can be considered a more accurate measure of the individual's speed of reaction in general than any single measurement. By way of analogy, in ice-skating, the marks of nine judges are combined, albeit in a somewhat complex way, into a single overall mark – you will be able to think of many other situations in sport and other contexts where this sort of procedure is followed.

Another example, to be dealt with in more detail below, is the derivation of an IQ score as a complex overall summary of performance on a variety of tasks.

THE IDEA OF A VARIABLE

In thinking about data, the notion of a *variable* is absolutely central. The term refers to any aspect of interest that varies (hence the name) among people, animals, or other units of analysis (for example, countries). Thus, we can conceive of *aggressiveness* as something that a person, an animal, or a country possesses to a greater or lesser degree.

In determining what counts as a variable, culture plays a major role. In particular, we tend to attribute the status of variable to any quality that has a name. Indeed, new names may be invented for this purpose – either in the wider culture, such as the relatively recent term 'male chauvinism', or within a more specialised scientific field, as in the less recent introduction of the introversion/extraversion dimension in psychology.

There is a very strong psychological tendency, once something is accepted implicitly as a variable, to assume that it has strong structural properties. Consider an abstract quality such as 'tolerance'. In the ways in which people talk about tolerance we may detect many implicit and debatable assumptions, in particular that:

(a) People differ in their level of tolerance.

(b) Each person can be considered to have, in some sense, a basic overall level of tolerance. Of course, it is recognised that this level is not constant over time, and is relative to target groups; for example, a person could be differentially tolerant in relation to race and religion (though these attitudes tend to be related).

(c) As a consequence, we are often prepared to make comments such as 'A is more tolerant than B'. More generally, the level of tolerance can be conceived as lying somewhere on a single dimension.

(d) The level of tolerance of each individual can be measured with some degree of precision and expressed as a single number.

There follow illustrative examples of variables and their associated measurement procedures.

HANDEDNESS

This is a simple example – but not as simple as you might think at first sight. It would be possible to simply ask each person 'Are you right-handed or left-handed?' but, in fact, handedness is not such a clear-cut matter. A person may be right-handed for some actions (opening a door, say), and left-handed for others (writing, say); or they may be ambidextrous. In practice, handedness is measured by means of a sample of behaviours. The *Edinburgh Handedness Inventory*, for example, asks the respondent to indicate if they have an absolute preference, or a preference for one hand or the other, or are indifferent, for activities such as writing and drawing, using tools and utensils, striking a match and so on. Foot and eye preference are also taken into account. The responses are used to determine a single score reflecting the degree of left- or right-handedness. (Note that this procedure assumes that a measure of handedness on a single dimension makes sense.)

REACTION TIME

Speed of reaction is of importance in many situations, including driving, and a considerable amount of research has been devoted to studying the factors that influence it. In the simplest experimental set-up, the participant waits for a stimulus to appear (a light coming on, say) and then makes a response as quickly as possible (by pressing a button, for example). Many more complex variants of this basic set-up may be used – for example, there may be several alternative stimuli and several alternative responses, and the participant is required to make a specific response corresponding to each specific stimulus. As already mentioned, repetitions of such a task typically show considerable variation in the measured reaction times for the same participant, so it is normal to average over a number of repetitions to obtain a more stable measure.

ATTITUDE TO COMPUTERS

It is very common to measure attitudes through questionnaires. By way of a specific example, one measure of attitudes to computers works in the following way. The respondent is asked to report his/her feelings by reacting to twenty statements such as:

Computers help people have easier lives

Computers help to create unemployment

The report is made by circling one of the numbers from 1 to 5 where:

1 = strongly agree

2 = agree

3 = undecided

4 = disagree

5 = strongly disagree.

For statements like the second cited above, the higher the number circled, the more positive the feeling reported. In this case, the numbers circled are added when calculating the total score. Conversely, for statements like the first, the higher the number circled, the more negative the feeling reported. In this case, the scale is reversed – 5 becomes 1, 4 becomes 2, and so on, for the purposes of calculating the total score. As a result, a total somewhere between 20 (the extreme negative response) and 100 (the extreme positive response) is obtained.

INTELLIGENCE

Tests of intelligence originated in France; but much of their subsequent development has taken place in the USA. The basic principle behind most such tests remains the sampling of a variety of tasks, each of which may be taken to require intelligence. More or less complex procedures are then used to score the component tasks and combine those scores into a single measure of IQ (you can easily find out details on specific IQ tests).

Beyond issues of what types of ability are indicative of intelligence, and what constitutes an adequate sample of the vast range of candidate tasks, there are deep controversies about the nature of intelligence testing, notably in relation to its cultural bias. Further, the assumption that it is appropriate to measure intelligence on a single dimension is itself controversial.

VARIABLES UNDER EXPERIMENTAL CONTROL

The above examples – handedness, reaction time, attitude to computers, and intelligence – are all cases where the value of the variable for any given person is inherent to that person, and not under the control of the experimenter. Such variables are called **subject variables** (although, given the trend away from using the term 'subject', they may well soon become known as **participant variables** – you heard it here first!). Socioeconomic status is one example. The researcher can select people for an experiment so that there are equal numbers of participants in different socioeconomic groups, but, for each individual participant, cannot decide what socioeconomic group that participant belongs to.

By contrast, there are experimental manipulations whereby participants can be assigned by the researcher to different values of a variable. For example, if an investigation is being carried out as to whether children perform better on a memory task if they are offered a reward for a good performance, then for each child tested, the researcher can decide which value of the dichotomous variable *reward/no reward* that child will take.

To illustrate the importance of **experimental control**, suppose a researcher wants to investigate the hypothesis that drinking coffee improves reaction time. Consider the differences between the following two approaches (presented in outline form without details).

Approach 1

Experimental participants turn up in the morning. The experimenter asks them if they drank coffee for breakfast. Their reaction times are measured subsequently and the values compared between the group of coffee-drinkers and the group of non-coffee-drinkers.

Approach 2

Experimental participants are asked not to drink coffee for 24 hours before the experiment. When they turn up for the experiment they are divided *randomly* into two groups. Here *randomly* means that any individual participant is equally likely to be assigned to either group – which could be done by tossing a coin, for example. The participants in one group are given two cups of coffee prior to having their reaction times measured, the other group do not drink any coffee.

BEFORE READING ON . . .

Think carefully about these two approaches. What implications do the differences between the approaches have for the interpretation of the data?

. . . now read on

There are many aspects to consider about these two approaches, but the key point we want to make here is the contrast between the researcher merely *measuring* the value of a variable (here the dichotomous variable coffee/no coffee) and being able to *control* the variable. This difference has a crucial importance when it comes to interpreting the results, even though the data will look exactly the same in the two cases.

Suppose the data suggest that coffee-drinkers do, in fact, have quicker reaction times. If these data have come from an experiment based on *Approach 1*, we cannot with total confidence attribute the difference to drinking coffee.

Student: Why not? It seems clear to me – if the coffee-drinkers have faster reaction times, it must be due to the coffee.

Lecturer: Well, here's one possible scenario. Let's just suppose that intelligence is related to coffee drinking – more intelligent people are more likely to drink coffee for breakfast. So when the participants turn up, and are divided into groups, the coffee-drinking group contains, in general, more intelligent people than the non-coffee-drinking group.

Student: So what?

Lecturer: Now suppose that intelligence is related to reaction time – the more intelligent you are, the faster your reaction time, in general. Do you get the point?

Student: Let's see. The coffee-drinking group is loaded with more intelligent people, according to your scenario, and they tend to have faster reaction times. And that's an alternative explanation for the difference in reaction times noted in the data.

Lecturer: Exactly! That's the point. We say that the samples of coffee-drinkers and non-coffee-drinkers are biased – in particular, if the postulated scenario holds good, they are biased with respect to intelligence, which may in turn be related to reaction time.

Student: OK, I'll buy that. So Approach 1 *isn't* a very good way to do an experiment, since you can't interpret the data with confidence?

Lecturer: That's right. Do you think Approach 2 *is* better?

Student: Well, I can see that randomly assigning participants to the two groups should mean that there would be no systematic differences between the two groups – in particular, they should be of about the same intelligence overall.

Lecturer: And the same goes for any other possible complicating factor. One of the important skills of being a good experimenter is designing your experiment so the story told by the data is not open to multiple interpretations.

The distinction highlighted in the above example, between simply measuring variables, as opposed to having them under experimental control, is a theme that recurs at many points in this book.

INVESTIGATING RELATIONSHIPS BETWEEN VARIABLES

Psychological research concerns itself with general questions of which the following are not untypical:

■ Do students with previous experience of using computers have more favourable attitudes towards them than those with no such previous experience?

■ Does coffee improve reaction time?

■ Do typists work faster in the morning than in the afternoon?

■ Is reaction time related to intelligence?

Each of these questions can be seen as a question about the relationship between two variables. In the first example, the two variables are:

■ attitude to computers; and

■ previous computer experience (a yes/no dichotomous variable).

The relationship between the two variables is investigated by comparing the attitude to computer scores between the two groups of participants – those with previous computer experience and those without. Note that previous computer experience is a *subject variable*, not under the control of the experimenter.

In the second example (assuming *Approach 2* as described above is used) the two variables are:

■ reaction time; and

■ consumption/non-consumption of coffee.

Again, the relationship between the two variables is investigated by comparing the reaction times between the two groups of participants. Here consumption/ non-consumption of coffee is under the control of the experimenter – an **independent variable**.

In the third example, let us assume that the approach adopted is to test a group of typists both in the morning and in the afternoon. The two variables are:

■ typing speed; and

■ time of day (morning/afternoon).

Note a major contrast with the first two examples. Here there is only one group of participants, each of whom is tested twice, and the comparison is *within* this group of participants, comparing their morning typing speeds and their afternoon typing speeds. The difference between comparisons made *between* groups of participants, and comparisons made *within* a single group of participants is another key distinction that will recur throughout this book.

In the final example, the two variables are:

- reaction time

- intelligence

Again, there is a contrast between this example and the preceding ones. Here, both variables are multi-valued, whereas in all the previous cases one of the variables was dichotomous. In this case, the question of interest is whether or not there is a relationship between reaction time and intelligence – is it the case that, in general, people with faster reaction times have higher intelligence; and, conversely, that people with slower reaction times have lower intelligence?

In each of these four examples, we are considering a possible relationship between two variables. Such a relationship cannot be observed directly. Instead, we must find some way to measure or assign each of the variables, so that data relating to the hypothesised relationship can be collected, and subjected to statistical analysis. The interpretation of this analysis then has implications for our view of the relationship between the variables.

Part I of this book shows how relationships between two variables of various types, including those illustrated in the four examples above, can be investigated through the design of appropriate experiments, the collection of data, and the statistical analysis of those data. In Part II, statistical methods for analysing more complex relationships between more than two variables are introduced.

CHAPTER REVIEW

In this chapter, we introduced, through examples, the key idea of variables as theoretical building-blocks, surveyed the types of variable experimental psychologists study, the procedures devised to measure these variables, and the nature of the numbers produced. The investigation of relationships between variables is central to psychological research.

Describing and summarising data

IN THIS
CHAPTER
. . .

. . . ways of organising a set of measurements for a group of participants on a single variable are set out. The first part deals with summary statistics; that is, numbers derived from the data that reflect important aspects of those data, namely averages and the amount of variation within the data set. Then a variety of graphical ways of displaying data is introduced.

SUMMARY STATISTICS

Below is a data set representing the scores of a class of 27 students on the *Attitude to Computers Scale* described in Chapter 2 (see page 24). The 27 numbers are initially written in no particular order.

```
60  62  62  47  63  69  68  46  70
60  56  54  48  50  49  58  49  66
54  53  56  52  57  63  71  61  43
```

An undigested list of numbers like this calls out for some organisation to bring out its salient features and patterns. We begin with numerical summaries, called *summary statistics*, before considering a variety of graphical methods for displaying the data set revealingly.

AVERAGES

The most familiar summary statistic is the *average*, as in figures such as the average number of children per married couple, average amount of rain in Manchester in June, average contents of a box of paperclips. In these cases, the average referred to is technically called the **mean**, which is calculated by adding all the cases and dividing by the number of cases. Note that, though 'average' is often taken to mean 'mean', it is a more general term, and there are several other types of average.

The total of the 27 *Attitude to Computers* scores listed above is 1547, which, when divided by 27, gives 57.3 (to one decimal place). (In passing, note that if you do this calculation on a calculator, you will get an answer like 57.296296 and, similarly, output from a statistical package may give the answer to many decimal places. In general, for values greater than 1, it is sufficient to round answers to one or, at most two, decimal places. For answers less than 1, three or, at most four significant figures – that is, digits other than leading zeros, will provide sufficient precision, for example, 0.573, 0.0573 . . .).

One way of thinking about the mean is as a point of balance (see Figure 3.1). If each number is thought of as a ball of standard weight placed on a (weightless) bar according to its value, then the mean is the point at which the configuration would be balanced.

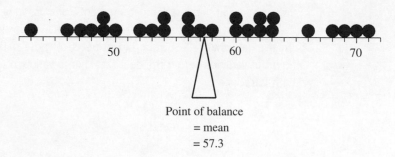

Point of balance
= mean
= 57.3

Figure 3.1 Mean as a point of balance

Another property of the mean is that if the differences between the individual scores and the mean (positive or negative) are worked out, then they balance out – that is, the sum of the positive differences and the sum of the negative differences are equal. In fact, this is why the balance model just illustrated works (think about it!).

Here's another example that may help to give you an intuitive feel for what 'the mean' means. Consider a group of five people varying in height, as indicated in Figure 3.2, which also shows where the mean height comes. Two people are above the mean height for the group and three are below. These differences above and below the mean balance out (check this numerically for yourself). If the people are thought of as acrobats standing on each others' heads, the total height is the same as it would be for another group of acrobats achieving the same feat, and consisting of quintuplets all equal in height to the mean of the first group.

The mean is just one form of average. For our purposes, of the other types there is one in particular that is important. It is called the **median**, and is calculated by ranking the measurements and taking the one that comes right in the middle. For example, if we rank the five people just discussed in terms of height, the median is the height of the one in the middle (see Figure 3.3). Note that it is different from the mean, though not by much in this case.

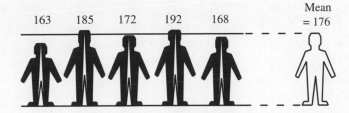

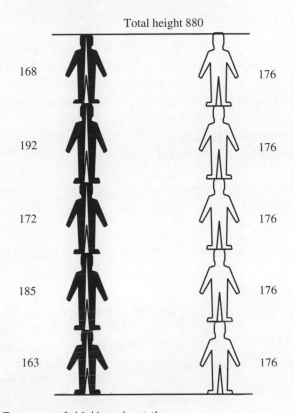

Figure 3.2 Two ways of thinking about the mean

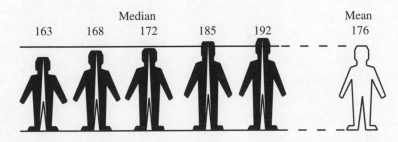

Figure 3.3 Median height of five people

BEFORE READING ON . . .

Find the median for the 27 *Attitude to Computers* scores listed on p. 29.

. . . now read on

It might occur to you to ask 'What if there are an even number of data, so there isn't *one* in the middle?' How do *you* think the procedure to calculate the median might be modified to take account of that? (The answer will be revealed later.)

Why is it helpful to have the median as an alternative to the mean? One reason is that it can be used with data that are simply ordered. Take the example of a teacher ranking the pupils in a class on mathematical ability. If you wanted to compare the girls and boys in the class, one way would be to work out the median (that is, middle rank) for the girls, and similarly for the boys.

There is an important reason for having the median available as an alternative to the mean, as illustrated by the following example.

Worker: My boss says the average salary in the company is £40 000 per year, but my union says the average salary is only £19 000. Who's lying?

Statistician: It's possible neither is lying.

Worker: I've heard the one about 'lies, damned lies, and statistics', but that's ridiculous.

Statistician: Let me explain. Your boss may be talking about one sort of average, and your union about another.

Worker: Go on.

Statistician: Let's suppose your boss pays himself £220 000 and the other eight workers £25 000, £22 000, £20 000, £19 000, £16 000, £15 000, £13 000, and £10 000. Add those all together and it comes to £360 000. Divide by 9 – the average is £40 000, as your boss says.

Worker: But that's not fair! He's the only one earning more than £40 000 – a lot more – and the rest of us are nowhere near £40 000.

Statistician: That's why your union chooses not to use the same average as your boss, which is called the mean (not because it is *mean*, though you might well consider it so).

Worker: So how does the union make it £19 000?

Statistician: They have used a different average, called the median. This is the one that comes in the middle when the numbers are put in order. You can see that it is £19 000. Most people would agree that this is a more sensible average to use in these circumstances – unlike the mean, it represents a more typical sort of salary in that firm, and it is not distorted by the anomalously high salary of the boss.

Worker: And they say figures can't lie!

Statistician: I prefer to put it this way – figures can't lie, but liars can figure. Remember that most statistics are presented by people with a vested interest in persuading you in one way or another. Even if you are not going to be a researcher, it's important that you know how to think critically about the statistics that you'll meet in your everyday life.

A single number within a set that is very different from most or all of the general run of numbers in that set – such as the boss's salary in that example – is called an **outlier** (of which more later). When a data set contains one or more outliers, it will often be more reasonable to use the median as an average rather than the mean.

One other average is commonly mentioned in statistics books (and thereafter ignored). For the sake of completeness, we shall do the same. It is called the **mode**, which is simply the value that occurs most often. It is not very useful, especially if you don't know how your scores are distributed, though for variables measured on a nominal scale, it can be considered as a rudimentary average.

The three averages we have introduced can be linked with scales of measurement as follows:

		Few/no outliers	Some/many outliers
nominal scale	<---------->	mode	mode
ordinal scale	<---------->	median	median
interval scale	<---------->	mean	median
ratio scale	<---------->	mean	median

MEASURING VARIATION

As summary statistics, averages are very useful. An average provides a single number that gives a general idea of the size of the numbers across the set as a whole. In particular, this makes it possible to make comparisons, and averages are very often used in this way in many contexts – education, business, sport, national characteristics and so on. However, an average has a major limitation, illustrated by the following example. If you are told the average temperature of a place over the year, this is not necessarily a good guide for deciding whether or not it is a good holiday destination – it could be that it is sometimes very hot and sometimes very cold, or it could be that it is moderately warm throughout the year, with little variation. There are a number of corny jokes on the same theme, such as the definition of a statistician as someone who thinks that if you stand with one foot in a bucket of boiling water and the other in a block of ice, then on average you are comfortable.

These examples remind us that, as well as an average, it is also usually essential to take into account how much the data vary. It is necessary, therefore, to have methods of quantifying the amount of **variation**, or **spread**, as it is sometimes called. A very simple way to do this is to calculate the **range**, which is just the difference between the highest and lowest values in the data set. However, you should be able to see that this is not a particularly sensible way of measuring spread, since it is based on only two values.

Instead, we consider two ways of measuring variation that reflect more of the information available in the data set. The first is called the **standard deviation**,

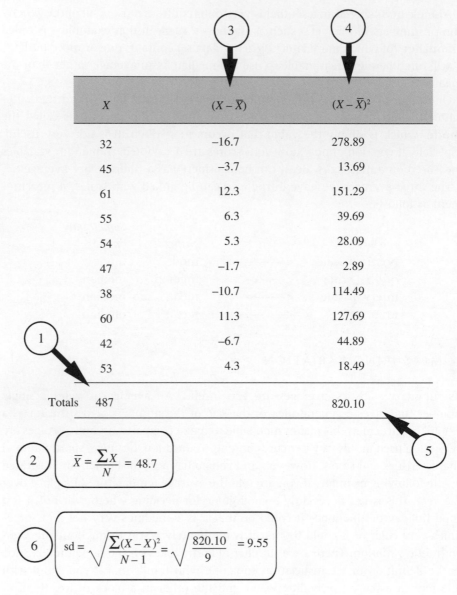

X	$(X - \bar{X})$	$(X - \bar{X})^2$
32	−16.7	278.89
45	−3.7	13.69
61	12.3	151.29
55	6.3	39.69
54	5.3	28.09
47	−1.7	2.89
38	−10.7	114.49
60	11.3	127.69
42	−6.7	44.89
53	4.3	18.49
Totals 487		820.10

$$\bar{X} = \frac{\sum X}{N} = 48.7$$

$$sd = \sqrt{\frac{\sum (X - X)^2}{N-1}} = \sqrt{\frac{820.10}{9}} = 9.55$$

Figure 3.4 Calculating the standard deviation

and Figure 3.4 presents a simple example to show how it is worked out for a set of ten numbers.

The steps in the calculation are as follows:

1. The first column contains the ten numbers, and 'X' stands for a general number in that set. The total of the numbers is 487.

2. $\sum X$ is standard notation meaning the *sum of all the X's* ($\sum$ being the Greek letter *sigma*, pronounced with the stress on the first syllable, corresponding to our S).

$\overline{X}$ is standard notation for the mean of the X scores, so the general formula for the mean is:

$$\overline{X} = \frac{\sum X}{N}$$

where N is the number of scores. The mean comes to 48.7 in this case.

3. Next, the mean is subtracted from each X score in turn, yielding sometimes a negative number and sometimes a positive number. $X - \overline{X}$ is called the **deviation from the mean**. As mentioned elsewhere, the sum of the deviations from the mean is, of necessity, zero.

4. Each deviation from the mean is squared.

5. The squared deviations are added, the total being 820.10 in this case.

6. The formula for standard deviation (sd) is:

$$sd = \sqrt{\frac{\sum (X - \overline{X})^2}{N - 1}}$$

leading to the value 9.55 for this example, as shown.

It should be clear that the standard deviation works as an overall measure of spread because it is based on how much the data points spread out around the central value represented by the mean. By squaring each deviation, dividing by $N - 1$, and then taking the square root, a sort of average of the deviations is obtained. (There are deep technical reasons that go beyond the scope of this book as to why this is considered an appropriate way to measure spread.)

One alternative way of measuring spread that we need to introduce is, analogously to the median, based on ranking procedures. For any set of data ranked in order of size, the **lower quartile** comes a quarter of the way along, and the **upper quartile** three-quarters of the way along (these definitions need to be made more precise, as you will see shortly). The **semi-interquartile range** (quite a mouthful, but reasonably self-explanatory) is half the difference between the upper and lower quartiles. Thus it is somewhat like the range, but not based on extreme values, so it is much better, since it will not be distorted by a single unusually large or small extreme value.

A quarter of the way along is too vague to specify how the calculation is actually done. Take these 11 numbers:

11, 13, 4, 2, 12, 15, 16, 7, 6, 3, 11

First arrange them in order from lowest to highest:

2, 3, 4, 6, 7, 11, 11, 12, 13, 15, 16

Now work out the 'location' of the lower quartile, which is given by the formula $\frac{1}{4}(N + 1)$, where N is the number of data points. That comes to 3 in this case, and

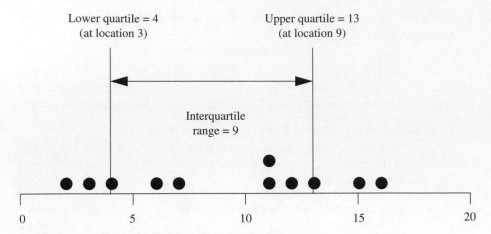

Figure 3.5 Quartiles and interquartile range (first example)

so the 3rd number along – which is 4 – is the lower quartile (see Figure 3.5). Similarly, the location of the upper quartile is given by $^3/_4(N + 1) = 9$, and so the upper quartile is 13. The semi-interquartile range is therefore $^1/_2(13 - 4) = 4.5$.

You may be wondering what happens if $^1/_4(N + 1)$ and $^3/_4(N + 1)$ do not conveniently turn out to be whole numbers. Suppose we add 19 to the previous set, so it is now:

2, 3, 4, 6, 7, 11, 11, 12, 13, 15, 16, 19

The formula for the location of the lower quartile now gives 3.25 – what does this mean as a location? Reasonably enough, a location of 3.25 is taken to mean a quarter (.25) of the way along from the third number towards the fourth number (see Figure 3.6). Since the third number is 4 and the fourth number is 6, this comes to 4.5, since the difference between 4 and 6 is 2, and .5 is a quarter of this. Similarly, you should be able to see that the upper quartile is 14.5 now, and so the semi-interquartile range is $^1/_2(14.5 - 4.5) = 5.0$ for the expanded data set.

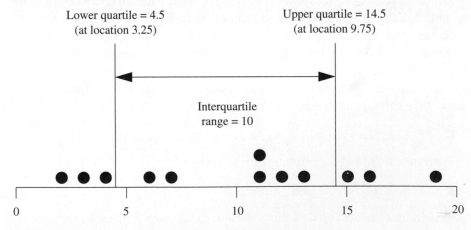

Figure 3.6 Quartiles and interquartile range (second example)

Remember we asked you earlier how you would calculate the median for a set of data with an even number of data points? What you do in such a case is to define the median as midway between the *two* middle scores. This is precisely equivalent to defining the location for the median by the formula $\frac{1}{2}(N + 1)$, whether N is odd or even (you should check that out to your satisfaction).

More generally, we can calculate **percentiles**. Roughly speaking, the kth percentile is such that in the data set, k per cent of the data are less than it and the remaining $(100 - k)$ per cent greater. To be precise, the formula for the location of the kth percentile is $\frac{k}{100}(N + 1)$ and the number corresponding to this is worked out in the same way as in the examples for the quartiles. If you think about it, lower quartile, median and upper quartile are other names for the 25th, 50th and 75th percentiles, respectively. Percentiles are useful for gauging where a particular score lies in relation to the set of scores as a whole. For example, if you were told that your mark of 67 in a statistics test was at the 94th percentile for the class, you would know that, roughly speaking, 6 per cent of the class scored higher and 94 per cent lower than you in the test.

Figure 3.7 summarises the four main summary statistics. The rank-based summary statistics share the property that they are not very much affected by outliers in the data set. For this reason, they are called **resistant** statistics. (An alternative term for the same idea that you may come across is **robust**.) By contrast, the mean and standard deviation are strongly affected by outliers, and so are called **non-resistant**. You will see that this theme of non-resistant statistics and alternative, rank-based resistant statistics recurs frequently in subsequent chapters.

	NON-RESISTANT	RESISTANT, RANK-BASED
AVERAGE	Mean	Median
MEASURE OF SPREAD	Standard deviation	Semi-interquartile range

Figure 3.7 Resistance of summary statistics

BEFORE READING ON . . .

The mean and median for the 27 *Attitude to Computers* scores listed on page 29 have already been calculated. Find the standard deviation and the semi-interquartile range for the same data set (use computer software or pencil-and-paper methods as you prefer). Now add three new numbers to the data set – 22, 23, 20 – and recalculate the four summary statistics. Look carefully at what happens.

. . . now read on

The exercise above shows that the addition of the three outliers has a big effect on the mean and standard deviation, but little effect on the median and semi-interquartile range, illustrating the point just made about non-resistant and resistant statistics.

GRAPHICAL REPRESENTATIONS OF DISTRIBUTIONS

Summary statistics are useful, but even an average and a measure of spread together give limited information about the distribution of data in the set as a whole. Graphical representations are valuable for examining the data set in more detail and making its main features salient, and statistical software should offer a range of these representations. Figures 3.8–3.11 illustrate several alternative ways of displaying the data set of 27 *Attitude to Computers* scores.

Dot plot

This simply plots a point along an axis for each of the numbers in the data set. The mean, median, standard deviation and interquartile range have been added here. Note that it makes sense to think of the mean and median as **points**, but the standard deviation and semi-interquartile range as **intervals**. One rough rule of thumb is that the standard deviation will tend to be about one-and-a-half times

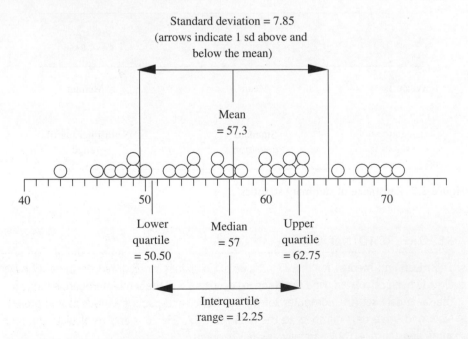

Figure 3.8 Dot plot of *Attitude to Computers* scores

as big as the semi-interquartile range. Another is that about $^2/_3$ of the scores will usually lie within 1 standard deviation of the mean (and about 95 per cent within two standard deviations).

Bar chart (or histogram)

The axis is divided into a number of intervals and the number (frequency) of data falling in each interval is represented by a column of the corresponding height. The columns collectively show the 'shape' of the distribution. You will also see this graph referred to as a **histogram**, which strictly is incorrect, since, in a histogram, frequency is represented by the *area* of the bars, rather than their height. This only becomes problematic in the rare instances where class intervals (given by the width of the bars) are not equal. In the vast majority of cases where class intervals are equal (as in our example), the height and area of the bars are directly proportional and, therefore, the shape of the graph will be the same regardless of whether height or area has been used to represent frequency. For this reason, we tend to prefer using the term 'bar chart' to refer to frequency graphs of discrete categories of data, such as males and females, or various faculties, and 'histogram' for continuous data divided into equal class intervals.

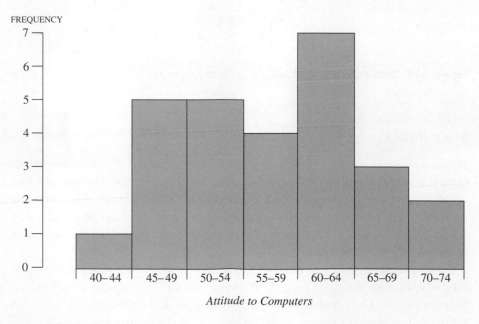

Figure 3.9 Histogram of *Attitude to Computers* scores

Stem-and-leaf

This is a quick pencil-and-paper method. Each number in the data set is split into two parts, *stem* and *leaf*. In the case of 2-digit numbers, as here, it's obvious how to do that – if there are more than 2 digits you would round to the first 2 or 3. The stems are presented vertically – here an extra feature has been introduced to spread the data out more, in that each of the stems has been subdivided. 4* is used for the range 40–44, and 4• for 45–49, and so on. The leaves are then placed, in order, opposite their stems. The shape of the distribution is again shown – in fact, the stem-and-leaf is rather like a histogram turned through a right-angle, with the added advantage that more information on the data is retained. Another advantage is that the data are ordered, making it easy to determine, say, the median.

7 *	0 1
6 •	6 8 9
6 *	0 0 1 2 2 3 3
5 •	6 6 7 8
5 *	0 2 3 4 4
4 •	6 7 8 9 9
4 *	3

Figure 3.10 Stem-and-leaf plot of *Attitude to Computers* scores

Box-and-whisker

This is a more complex graphical summary of the distribution. The 'box' extends from the lower quartile to the upper quartile, with the median marked as a line within it. From each end of the box a **whisker** is drawn, the top one extending up to the 90th percentile and the bottom one down to the 10th percentile. Any points lying beyond these limits are plotted individually. (Note that the definition of the whiskers is different in some computer packages.)

If you add the three extra data – 22, 23, 20 – to any of these representations they will show up clearly as outliers. To check that you understand the procedure for constructing a box-and-whisker plot, we suggest you do that for the enlarged set of 30 data (and compare it with the one for the 27 data).

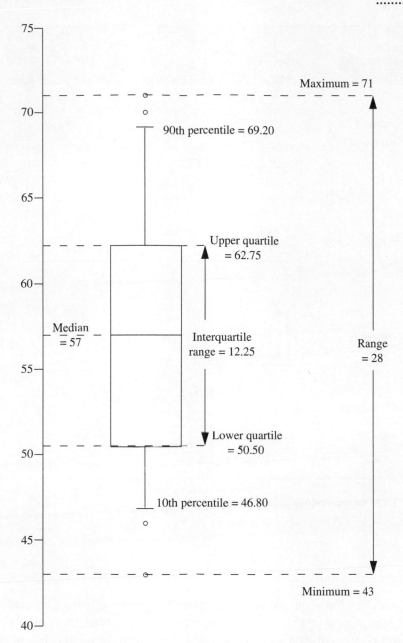

Figure 3.11 Box-and-whisker plot of *Attitude to Computers* scores

SHAPES OF DISTRIBUTIONS

As mentioned, histograms in particular are useful in displaying the shape of a distribution. A number of general shapes may be distinguished, as indicated in Figure 3.12. In each case, a typical histogram is shown, together with a schematic indication of the general shape.

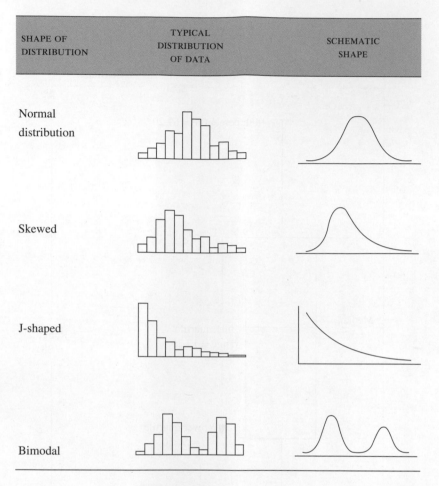

Figure 3.12 Various shapes of distribution

The normal distribution

Many variables found in psychological research produce distributions conforming, at least approximately, to this shape (sometimes called the **Bell Curve**). Graphical displays of data showing physical characteristics such as height often conform very closely to this shape. Intelligence is assumed to be distributed in the same way and measures of intelligence are scaled accordingly.

Skewed

This shape is like a normal distribution that has been stretched out more at one end than the other. Reaction times tend to produce this sort of shape – there is clearly a lower limit (zero, ultimately) but no upper limit, and in any set of reaction times there may be some that are high relative to the rest.

J-shaped

In this case, values taper off very quickly. An example of a variable that would tend to yield such a distribution is the number of accidents in a year for workers in a factory, in which case most of the workers might well have 0, some would have 1, and the frequencies would tail off quickly thereafter. (The shape is supposed to resemble a reflected letter J.)

Bimodal

Here the distribution has two 'peaks' when represented as a histogram, indicating relative concentrations of frequencies at two separate places on the scale ('mode' in this context refers to high points in the histogram). This sort of shape is relatively rare. An example would be handedness, where people tend to be either predominantly left-handed or predominantly right-handed (there are more of the latter).

An important general point to understand is how the various shapes of distribution reflect the nature of the variable whose data are being displayed. Many characteristics of people naturally lead to a normal distribution (at least approximately) but, as examples above show, there are other variables which equally naturally lead to very different shapes of distribution.

CHAPTER REVIEW

In this chapter, summary statistics – numbers derived from the data reflecting salient aspects of the data – were introduced. We began with two sorts of average, mean and median, with discussion of when the median is a more sensible option. Similarly, two measures of spread, standard deviation and semi-interquartile range, were defined. It was stressed that the median and semi-interquartile range are resistant (robust) by comparison with the mean and standard deviation, in that outliers have a much weaker effect on them.

In the second part of the chapter, a variety of graphical means for displaying sets of data for a single variable were illustrated. We pointed out the logical relationship between the nature of a variable and the shape of the distribution of scores that it typically produces.

4 Seeing patterns in data: Comparing

IN THIS CHAPTER
. . .

. . . ways of organising and displaying data to reveal important patterns are shown. All the examples in this chapter are about making comparisons between two sets of measurements, using data taken from samples of people. In this way, it is possible to investigate empirically questions such as:

■ Do Arts and Science students differ in their preferences for various courses in psychology?

■ Do squash players react more quickly than chess players?

■ Does drinking coffee improve speed of reaction?

A key point of the chapter is that data from samples can only offer evidence in relation to such questions, not definitive answers.

COMPARING PROPORTIONS

HINT, HINT

One of the Gestalt psychologists who studied problem-solving more than fifty years ago was N.R.F. Maier. Figure 4.1 is based on one of the problems he investigated. Can you see a solution?

One line of investigation is to see whether a hint would help participants find the solution. Accordingly, for half the participants tested, the experimenter contrives to brush against one of the hanging strings to set it swinging. For the other half, this hint is not given. (The solution – or, at least, *one* solution – to the problem is to tie the hammer to one of the strings, set it swinging, hold the other string and wait for the hammer to swing close enough to be grabbed.) Accordingly, data

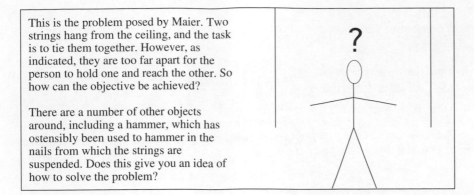

This is the problem posed by Maier. Two strings hang from the ceiling, and the task is to tie them together. However, as indicated, they are too far apart for the person to hold one and reach the other. So how can the objective be achieved?

There are a number of other objects around, including a hammer, which has ostensibly been used to hammer in the nails from which the strings are suspended. Does this give you an idea of how to solve the problem?

Figure 4.1 The Maier problem

in the four cells of a 2 × 2 table can be collected and might look like those in Figure 4.2.

Note that the table shows a relationship between two variables of a simple type not considered previously, in which both variables are dichotomous. The variable *without hint/with hint* is under the control of the experimenter through, for example, random assignment of participants to the levels.

	NO. OF SUCCESSES	NO. OF FAILURES
WITHOUT HINT	15	25
WITH HINT	31	9

Figure 4.2 2 × 2 frequency table – Maier data

BEFORE READING ON . . .

Do *you* think that these data would prove that a hint helps to solve the problem? Think carefully about how you would justify your answer to someone who was sceptical about this conclusion.

. . . now read on

More participants in the group given the hint solved the problem (31 out of 40) than in the group not given the hint (15 out of 40). That is clear. Expressed in percentage terms, the difference is 78 per cent as against 38 per cent. (Note: the exact percentages are 77.5 per cent and 37.5 per cent but we shall generally round percentages to the nearest percentage, rounding up if it's a case of .5.)

Person in street: So, it has been proved that giving the hint helps people to solve the problem.

Statistician: It depends what you mean by 'proved'. Nineteen people who were given the hint still didn't solve the problem, and fifteen people who weren't given the hint did.

Person in street: OK, what I mean is that people given the hint are more likely to solve the problem.

Statistician: Do you think everyone is equally good at solving problems in general, or this one in particular?

Person in street: No, clearly some people are smarter than others. For example, I can solve crosswords quickly, but I know many people who can't do them at all.

Statistician: So, some people would solve Maier's problem easily, while at the other extreme, some would never get it?

Person in street: Yes.

Statistician: What if, by chance, the people Maier put in the hint group were mostly smart, while those in the no-hint group were mostly poor at solving problems? Wouldn't that be an alternative explanation for the results?

Person in street: I see what you mean. But that's unlikely to happen. By the law of averages, since he assigned people randomly to groups, the two groups are bound to be of the same overall level of smartness.

Statistician: Ah, if only I had a pound – or a dollar – for every time the law of averages was appealed to without true understanding of what it means. It's true that there is a good chance that the groups will be roughly equal in smartness, but there remains the possibility that they are not.

Person in street: So, why bother doing an experiment if you can't reach conclusions when you've got the data?

Statistician: It's not as bad as that. The data strongly support the hypothesis that giving the hint helps. But we cannot say that they prove it. See the difference?

Person in street: Okay, but aren't you being vague? Just how strong is the evidence in support of the theory?

Statistician: That is a very complex and controversial issue. Statistical theory has a number of suggested procedures to lend more precision to such statements, and this is mostly what statistics books are about.

A QUESTION OF TASTE

In a psychology course, all students in two faculties were asked to nominate their favourite among four modules given in one session – Psycholinguistics, Social Psychology, Statistics, Human–Computer Interaction (HCI). The collated data are as shown in Figure 4.3.

	PSYCHOLINGUISTICS	SOCIAL	STATS	HCI	TOTAL
ARTS	27	35	3	8	73
SCIENCE	13	9	3	18	43

Figure 4.3 Frequency table (*Faculty* × *Favourite Module*)

Here the two variables being related are *Favourite Module* (on a nominal scale, with four values) and *Faculty* (dichotomous). Faculty is an example of what we defined in Chapter 2 as a subject variable.

BEFORE READING ON . . .

Study the data and note down the main points of interest.

. . . now read on

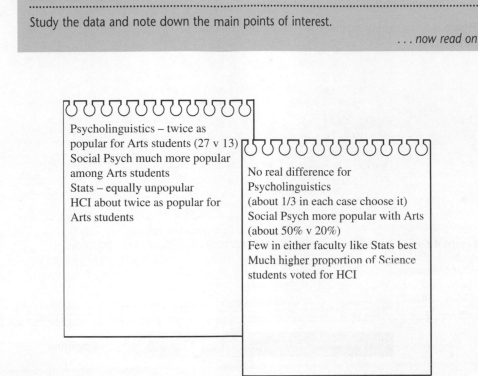

Figure 4.4 Two interpretations of *Favourite Module* data

Compare the notes made by two students, shown in Figure 4.4. We hope it is clear to you that the second student's interpretation is much more sensible. Remember the old riddle: why do white sheep produce more wool than black sheep? Because there are more of them! Where the total numbers differ, proportional rather than absolute numbers are more helpful for making comparisons. Following the second student's lead, the data can be converted systematically to percentages, as shown in Figure 4.5.

Instead of a table of percentages, various graphical devices are available for making patterns in the data visible to the eye, including pie charts, strip charts and composite bar charts (see Figures 4.6–4.8).

Of the various tabular and graphical representations shown, which do you think is easiest to use? Indeed, maybe *you* could invent a better way of showing the data.

	PSYCHOLINGUISTICS	SOCIAL	STATS	HCI	TOTAL
ARTS	37%	48%	4%	11%	100%
SCIENCE	30%	21%	7%	42%	100%

Figure 4.5 Percentage table (*Faculty × Favourite Module*)

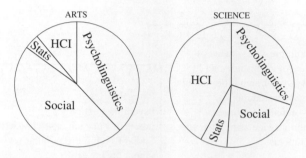

Figure 4.6 Pie charts (*Faculty × Favourite Module*)

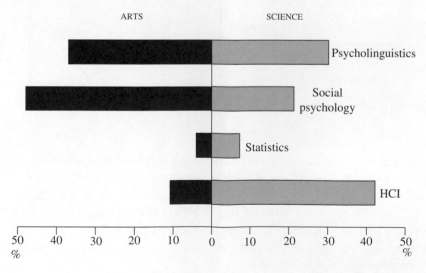

Figure 4.7 Strip chart (*Faculty × Favourite Module*)

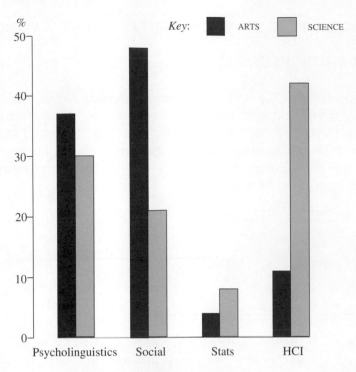

Figure 4.8 Composite histogram (*Faculty* × *Favourite Module*)

Student: I thought the table was easiest to use and interpret, but my friend preferred the composite histogram.

Statistician: Well, there is no 'right answer' here. People differ in their preferences.

Student: Anyway, however you look at them, the results are clear here. All the students were tested, so there is no sample involved.

Statistician: That's true. If you are only interested in these students in their own right, then the results seem pretty clear-cut – but not entirely.

Student: Why not? It seems pretty cut-and-dried to me.

Statistician: Well, consider this, for example. If the students were tested again three months later,

mightn't at least some of them have changed their opinions?

Student: That is possible, but it seems unlikely that more that a few would.

Statistician: Fair enough. Notice, by the way, how often you are using words such as likely and unlikely in our discussions. Now, here is another major point. Suppose the focus is not on this class of students specifically, but on Arts and Science students in general – for simplicity, let's confine it to the single university in question.

Student: Let me anticipate you here. If the survey was done the next year, the results might be different.

Statistician: You've got it! It's the same message again. The data are suggestive – maybe very suggestive – but not conclusive.

COMPARISON BETWEEN INDEPENDENT SAMPLES

QUICK ON THE DRAW

Squash is a fast game. The ball travels at very high speeds, giving players fractions of a second to make decisions and carry out complex motor movements. By contrast, chess players may take as long as an hour thinking about a single move (although under time pressure, fast thinking and moving may become decisive). It is plausible to conjecture that squash players may have faster reaction times than chess players, on the grounds that:

only people with fast reaction times will play squash

OR

playing squash improves reaction time

OR

a combination of the above and other explanations.

To investigate the question experimentally, reaction times for groups of participants from a squash club and from a chess club were measured. The data are as shown in Figure 4.9.

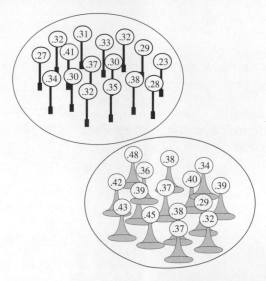

Figure 4.9 *Quick on the draw* – reaction times (seconds) for squash and chess players

BEFORE READING ON . . .

Do these data support the hypothesis that squash players have faster reaction times than chess players? How could you display the data to make a visual comparison easy?

. . . now read on

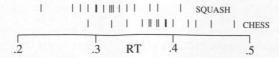

Figure 4.10 Multiple line plots for *Quick on the draw* data

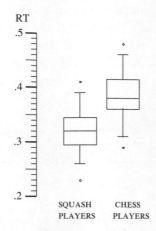

Figure 4.11 Box-and-whisker plots for *Quick on the draw* data

	SQUASH		CHESS
		.4*	5 8
	1	.4•	0 2 3
	8 7 5	.3*	6 7 7 8 8 9 9
4 3 2 2 2 1 0 0		.3•	2 4
	9 8 7	.2*	9
	3	.2•	

Figure 4.12 Back-to-back stem-and-leaf plots for *Quick on the draw* data

A variety of graphical representations, involving extensions of methods introduced in Chapter 3, can be used to provide visual comparisons between those on the court and those on the board (see Figures 4.10–4.12). Consider each graphical representation in turn. What specific features of each one suggest that, overall, squash players do have quicker reaction times?

A complementary approach is to calculate and compare averages.

	MEAN	MEDIAN
Squash players	.32	.32
Chess players	.39	.38

BEFORE READING ON . . .

Look back to the graphical representations of the data. Note where the mean and median for each group are located on these graphs.

. . . *now read on*

Figure 4.13 shows yet another way to look at the data. Are the faster people predominantly squash players and the slower ones chess players? A simple way to get a handle on this is to rank them. The three fastest times are .23 (squash player); .27 (squash player); .28 (squash player); and then come a squash player and a chess player tying on .29. Continuing the analysis leads to the sequence:

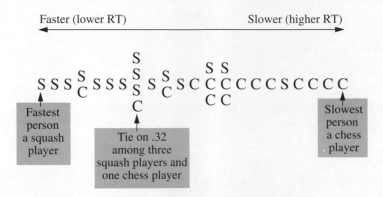

Figure 4.13 Combined ranking of squash and chess players' scores

Squash player: *That looks pretty conclusive to me. Although not all the squash players are faster than all the chess players, the trend is clear. The faster ones are mostly our guys and the slower ones are the pawn-pushers.*

Statistician: *I agree. There's a remote technical possibility that very unrepresentative samples were picked, but the data look very strong.*

WHAT IF?

What if two more squash players had been tested and their reaction times were .55 seconds and .58 seconds? These wayout data could arise in a number of ways. If it is decided to take them seriously, then each of the graphical representations can be amended accordingly, as in Figures 4.14–4.16. Note how the two extra data stand out like sore thumbs. Consider also the effect on the mean. Revised to take account of the two new data, the mean for the squash players becomes .36,

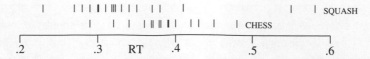

Figure 4.14 Multiple line plots of squash and chess scores (with outliers)

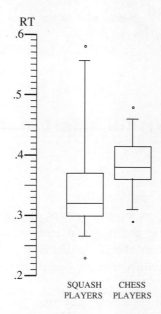

Figure 4.15 Box-and-whisker plots of squash and chess scores (with outliers)

SQUASH		CHESS
8 5	.5*	
	.5•	
	.4*	5 8
1	.4•	0 2 3
8 7 5	.3*	6 7 7 8 8 9 9
4 3 2 2 2 1 0 0	.3•	2 4
9 8 7	.2*	9
3	.2•	

Figure 4.16 Back-to-back stem-and-leaf plots of squash and chess scores (with outliers)

which is only marginally faster than the mean of .39 for the chess players. Would it make sense, in that case, to conclude that there is really no evidence for a difference between the groups? By contrast, adding new data generally has a small effect on the median, and, in fact, in this case it doesn't change it at all! (Check this out for yourself to see why.)

Squash player: These two extra guys have really let us down. Couldn't we just ignore them? Obviously the apparatus was faulty, or they didn't understand the instructions, or they weren't paying attention. Surely you can't take them seriously!

Statistician: The technical name for such data is outliers. When a few really wayout data like this occur,

it's right to be careful. First, it should be considered whether something did go wrong that would legitimise ignoring these data as mavericks. That is one possible course of action. Another is to use a different statistic that is resistant, namely not so markedly affected by outliers. In this case, it can be argued that the median is preferable to the mean if comparison of averages is to be used.

COMPARISON WITHIN PAIRED DATA

COFFEE TIME

Whether coffee quickens reaction time can be tested experimentally. One approach would be to set up separate groups of participants, and test reaction times for both groups. One group would receive coffee and the other group would not. In such a situation, the group that is treated in some way is generally called the **experimental group**, and the group not treated is called the **control group**.

An alternative approach is to use just one group of people, but to test each person in the group on two occasions, once with and once without coffee. The contrast between the two approaches is shown schematically in Figure 4.17.

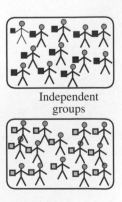

Independent groups

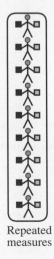

Repeated measures

Figure 4.17 Two approaches to experimentation – independent groups and repeated measures. Each little 'box' represents one piece of data.

BEFORE READING ON . . .

What advantages can you think of for the second approach? And what disadvantages?

. . . now read on

The second experimental design is more incisive, in general. This is because it compares the same individuals under the two conditions, rather than unrelated people. On the other hand, care should be taken to make sure when this experimental design is used that the testing of an individual on the first occasion does not affect their performance on the second occasion – unlikely, in this case.

Figure 4.18 presents some data for such an experiment. They could be displayed using one of the representations introduced earlier, such as a back-to-back stem-and-leaf plot. However, there is a major drawback of such a representation in that it loses important information in the data, namely which *with-coffee* measurement is linked with which *without-coffee* measurement. Figure 4.19 gives an alternative representation which retains that information; we call this a **related line chart**.

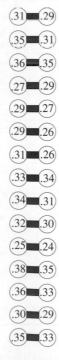

Figure 4.18 *Coffee time* data – repeated measures (reaction time in seconds)

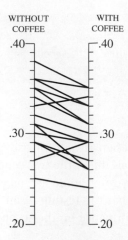

Figure 4.19 Graphical display of repeated measures data (*Coffee time*)

BEFORE READING ON . . .

If a linking line slopes up from left to right, what does it mean?
If a linking line slopes down from left to right, what does this mean?

. . . now read on

If the line slopes up, it means that the RT with coffee is higher; that is, the person whose two measurements are represented by that line was slower with coffee than without. Conversely, if the line slopes down, it means the *with-coffee* RT was faster.

Figure 4.20 shows another possible way to show the data. Each individual tested has two measures – RT without coffee and RT with coffee. Each such pair of data

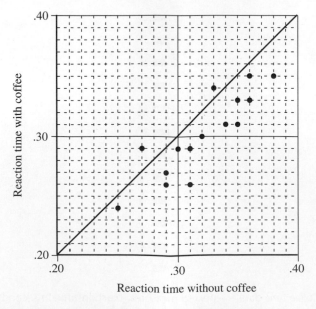

Figure 4.20 Alternative graphical display of *Coffee time* data

can be represented by a point on a two-dimensional graph, with RT without coffee on the horizontal axis and RT with coffee on the vertical axis. The collection of such points gives an overall picture of the data. Note that a diagonal line has been added, which passes through all the points in the plane where RT without coffee and RT with coffee would be the same.

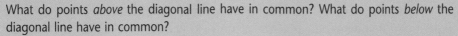

BEFORE READING ON . . .

What do points *above* the diagonal line have in common? What do points *below* the diagonal line have in common?

. . . now read on

The diagonal line passes through all the points of equality for the two measurements. A point above the diagonal line corresponds to an individual with a higher RT with coffee than without, and a point below the diagonal line corresponds to an individual with a lower RT with coffee. Moreover, the further any point is from the diagonal line, the bigger the difference between the two RTs, in one direction or another.

A different approach is to carry out a pair-by-pair comparison. As a simple first step, count the number of cases where the person performed faster with coffee and the number where the person performed slower with coffee. In fact, you can do this directly from either of the graphical representations – there are 13 of the former type, and 2 of the latter.

All of the representations tell a consistent story. For the sample of participants tested, in most cases, reaction time is faster after coffee.

Person in street: But there were two people who performed less well with coffee. Maybe the world is made up of two sets of people – those whose reaction times are speeded up by coffee, and those whose reaction times are slowed down.

Statistician: That is possible. In that case, the data provide some support for the hypothesis that the former type is more frequent. There are other possibilities though. It could be, for example, that the two people who were slower with coffee just happened to have unusually slow reactions for some of those particular trials. Remember that there will always be variation in reaction times measured repeatedly for the same individual.

ON NOT JUMPING TO CONCLUSIONS

In all of the above cases, it should be clear that the data presented offer evidence for judging the questions posed, suggesting that:

- hints help people to solve problems;

- there are marked preferences for certain subjects over others among psychology students, and the patterns differ for Arts and Science students;

- squash players have faster reactions times than chess players; and

- coffee speeds up reaction time.

At the same time, it has been pointed out repeatedly that absolute, cut-and-dried answers are not forthcoming. The main reason for this is the fact that the data are only a sample of all the possible data. For example, in the problem-solving experiment involving hanging strings, only 80 people were tested. Let's suppose these 80 people were first-year university students. Then there is a much larger group of all first-year university students, even if we restrict it to the country in which the study was carried out. Moreover, the potential pool of experimental participants would be widened even more if first-year students over many years were included. The technical term for such a potential pool, however defined, is **population**. Experiments of this sort, therefore, are based on testing a **sample** from a very much larger population, with the hope of being able to make general statements about the population on the basis of the sample.

Thus, on the basis of the data described, it would be reasonable to state a conclusion such as 'there is some evidence that hints can help people to solve problems'. However, caution is needed. Not only have we data restricted to a sample of the target population, but it also only relates to one particular hint and one particular problem. Similar experiments would be needed with other problems and other hints to build up a general picture. Only if a consistent trend emerged would we justified in making a general statement about the efficacy of hints in problem-solving.

Similar cautionary remarks apply to the other examples. In Chapter 7, we shall start to show some approaches that give a handle on the general problem of **statistical inference**, namely the making of inferences about populations on the basis of data for samples.

COMPARISONS AS RELATIONSHIPS BETWEEN VARIABLES

The examples discussed above fit into the general framework described in Chapter 2, of relationships between variables. They have in common also that at least one of the variables in each case is dichotomous; that is, has only two values. For this reason, the relationship between the variables in each of these cases can be explored by comparisons between two sets of data. In the next chapter, by contrast, we consider relationships between variables, both of which take multiple values.

CHAPTER REVIEW

This chapter has presented examples of ways of looking at data:

■ Comparing percentages of responses from different groups.
Example: *Do the percentages of students preferring various courses differ between two faculties?*

■ Comparing two groups' measurements on some variable.
Example: *Do squash players tend to have faster reaction times than chess players?*

■ Comparing performances of one group of people under different conditions.
Example: *Do people react more quickly after drinking coffee than without coffee?*

Throughout the chapter, the absolutely central point has been stressed that data for a sample does not offer an absolute answer to any experimental question about a general population. Data for a sample must always be considered against the background of what might have been.

5 Seeing patterns in data: Correlating

IN THIS
CHAPTER
. . .

. . . more ways of organising and displaying data to reveal important patterns are shown. Whereas Chapter 4 was about relationships between variables in terms of *comparisons* between two sets of data, this chapter deals with relationships between two variables, bearing on such questions as:

- Is it generally true that the taller someone is, the heavier they are?

- Is it true that people's intelligence relates to the size of their head?

- Do tests that are intended to measure the same variable present a consistent picture?

- Does academic performance reduce as the number of parties attended by students increases?

As in the previous chapter, it is emphasised how data from a sample can only offer degrees of evidence in addressing these questions, and not definitive answers.

THE CONCEPT OF CORRELATION

Proverbial wisdom has it that 'the bigger they come, the harder they fall' and 'more haste, less speed'. Whether or not these are generally true, there are very many situations that can be characterised in the form *the more of A, the more of B* or, conversely *the more of A, the less of B*. For example, it is accepted that the richer people are, the more conservative they are politically. Of course, this is just an overall trend, since we can think of rich people with left-wing views, and poor people with right-wing views. Similarly, in general – but by no means universally – the more education you have, the more you will earn.

Within psychology, there is a large number and variety of situations in which the relationship between two variables is of interest. A selection of illustrative examples follows.

A MATTER OF OPINION

Social psychologists are interested in postulated personality traits such as authoritarianism and conservatism. One form of evidence in support of such claims is when stated opinions can be shown to be related. For example, supporting harsher sentences for criminals and supporting corporal punishment in schools might both be considered indicative of authoritarianism. Figure 5.1 presents a set of possible data relating to this question in the form of a 2 × 2 table. It can be seen that more of those tested either support both views or oppose both views than support one and oppose the other. These data therefore represent some evidence for the hypothesis that the views are related, and the underlying hypothesis that there is a trait accounting for this relationship.

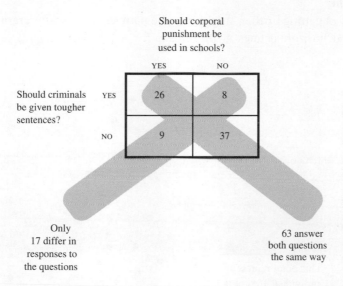

Figure 5.1 2 × 2 frequency table – sentencing and corporal punishment data

Person in street: So what? People who want to punish criminals want to punish schoolchildren. I could have told you that.

Social psychologist: Bear in mind that this is just a small example to illustrate how we build up a picture of a theoretical construct such as authoritarianism. These data are just one piece of the jigsaw that allows us to theorise about the nature of authoritarianism and the ways in which it is manifested – some of which are not obvious – as well as providing ways of measuring the strength of the trait as it differs from individual to individual.

HEIGHT AND WEIGHT

Whereas the previous example was about the relationship between variables taking only two values, this one is about the relationship between two variables measured on a continuous scale. The data are for 60 male psychology students. To investigate the relationship between the two variables, an excellent graphical resource is to hand (see Figure 5.2). For each student in the sample, there are two data – height and weight. Each such pair of measurements can be represented by a single point on a two-dimensional graph, where height is measured on the horizontal axis and weight on the vertical axis. A complete display of all such points for the sample is called a **scattergram** or **scatterplot**. In the scattergram you can see a trend whereby weight tends to be greater (but by no means always) if height is greater. A relationship of this sort is called a **positive correlation**.

One way of getting further insight into the pattern in the scattergram is to draw vertical and horizontal lines at the means for height and weight, respectively,

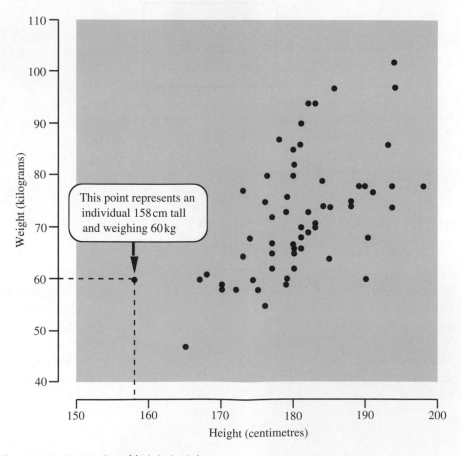

Figure 5.2 Scatterplot of height/weight

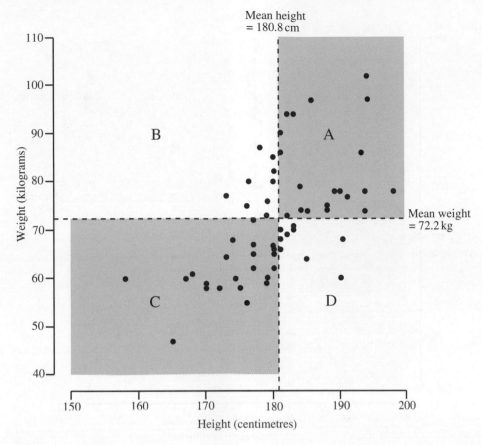

Figure 5.3 Height/weight scatterplot slowing quadrants

dividing the data into four quadrants, labelled A, B, C, D as in Figure 5.3. The points in quadrant A correspond to the individuals in the sample who are of above mean height and above mean weight. The points in quadrant B correspond to those of below mean height but above mean weight . . . and so on. The cases that fall in quadrants A and C are in line with the general trend that relatively tall people tend to be relatively heavy, and relatively short people tend to be relatively light; the less numerous cases in quadrants B and D correspond to the exceptions to the general trend who are smaller but heavier, or taller but lighter, respectively.

BIGHEADS

Does intelligence depend on the size of your head? Many people have thought so, including Paul Broca, a medical professor who founded the Anthropological Society of Paris in 1859. He firmly believed that intelligence depended on the size

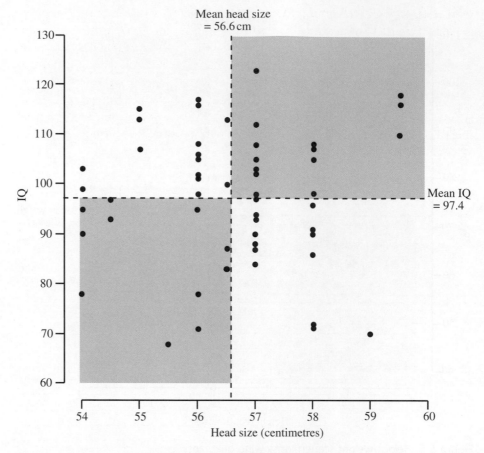

Figure 5.4 Head size/IQ scatterplot (with quadrants)

of the brain – hence, for example, men are more intelligent than women because their brains are larger.

The scatterplot in Figure 5.4 shows the data for 54 female psychology students. As you can see, there is no sign in these data of a relationship between size of head and measured intelligence. This lack of relationship is reflected in the fact that the points are evenly distributed among the four quadrants.

CONSISTENCY

As was discussed in Chapter 2, psychologists devote considerable time and ingenuity to devising ways of measuring postulated patterns of behaviour that can be described as variables, with assumptions that these can be measured on a single numerical scale. One of the examples of such a construction was a test for measuring attitudes towards computers. One way of evaluating whether such tests are appropriate is to see how much consistency there is between two such tests, each of which purports to measure a given variable. If the variable is a viable construct, and each of the tests does indeed measure it, then the results should be consistent – individuals scoring high on one test should also score high on the other, and individuals scoring low on one test should also score low on the other.

The scatterplot in Figure 5.5 shows data for a sample of 58 male students for two tests designed to measure their attitudes towards computers. As can be seen, there is an overall relationship between the two sets of scores, though the pattern is by no means perfect.

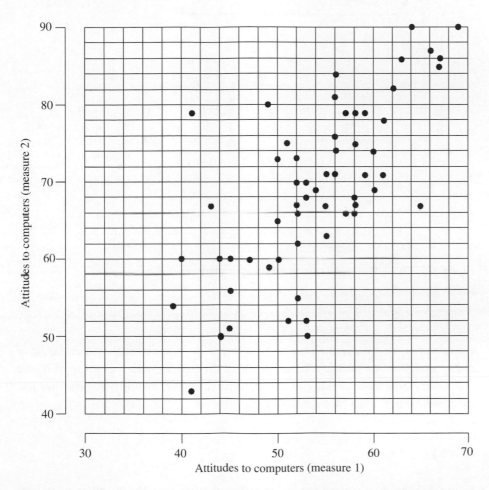

Figure 5.5 Scatterplot of two measures of computer attitudes

CRITICAL THINKING

Another example of using correlation to examine consistency is when the judgements of two people are considered to see how consistent they are. Figure 5.6 presents data on the rankings of three people of a selection of ten classic movies.

	A	B	C
Battleship Potemkin	6	5	9
Bicycle Thieves	5	3	6
The Birds	10	9	2
Casablanca	9	8	1
Citizen Kane	4	6	5
High Noon	8	10	7
If...	7	7	4
Jules et Jim	2	4	8
Pulp Fiction	3	1	3
Seven Samurai	1	2	10

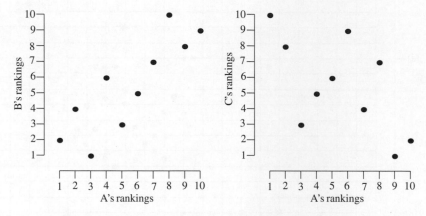

Figure 5.6 Classic film rankings and resulting scatterplots

Using scatterplots to examine the consistency, it becomes clear that A and B have rather similar views on the relative merits of the movies, whereas those of A and C are very different. Looking at the data in the table, would you say that the judgements of B and C are similar or not?

PARTY TIME

Figure 5.7 presents some data for thirty students about the number of parties attended during an academic year, and the average marks obtained at the end of that year. (These data are, of course, *entirely* fictitious.) From the scattergram, we see that there is an overall relationship whereby the greater the number of parties, in general, the lower the marks. When there is a relationship between two variables of this sort, with high scores on one variable tending to go with low ones on the other, it is called a **negative correlation**. Note how, in this case, the majority of the points lie in quadrants B and D.

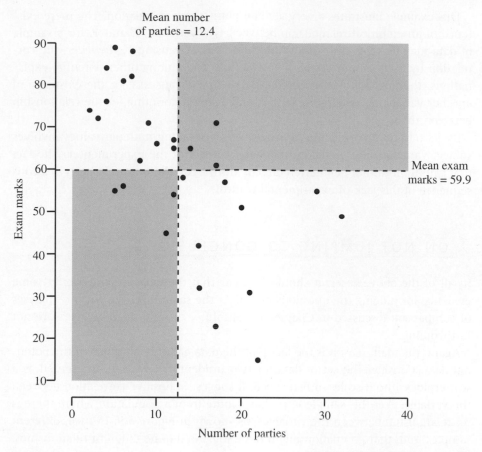

Figure 5.7 Negative correlation – party attendance and exam performance

CORRELATION AND CAUSATION

Suppose – for the sake of argument – that the last set of data presented for party-going and academic performance was authentic. What conclusions would be suggested by such data?

Student A: *It looks like going to parties causes you to do badly in your course. I can buy that. If you want to do well, cut down on socialising is the message.*

Student B: *That's one possible explanation, but I can think of others. It's a matter of personality. Some people are serious and work hard, others like to enjoy themselves.*

This is the underlying cause for both the amount of partying and the level of performance.

Student C: *Here's another theory. We all have a fair idea of how we're doing. Maybe the ones who know they aren't going to do well go to parties to cheer themselves up. So the level of performance influences the social behaviour, not the other way round.*

This example illustrates a very general point about correlation. The mere existence of an empirical relationship between two variables, X and Y, for a sample of data may be suggestive of a causal link, with X causing Y. However, the correlation by itself cannot establish such a link, and among other potential explanations, the possibility must be considered that Y causes X, or the existence of another variable Z, underlying both X and Y and accounting for the relationship between them.

By its nature, a correlation between variables taking multiple values involves subject variables, not variables under the control of the experimenter. The fact that causation cannot be inferred directly from a correlation can be seen as a consequence of this lack of experimental control.

ON NOT JUMPING TO CONCLUSIONS

In all of the above cases, it should be clear that the data presented offer some evidence for judging the questions posed. At the same time – as for the analyses of comparison discussed in Chapter 4 – absolute, cut-and-dried answers are not forthcoming.

Again, the main reason is the fact that the data are only a sample of the potential data. Consider the set of data for two unidentified variables presented as a scatterplot without scales in Figure 5.8. It suggests a positive correlation between the variables. Yet this sample *might* have come from a population where there is no relationship between the variables, as shown in Figure 5.9. In turn, different samples from that population might have suggested quite different relationships, even possibly a negative correlation.

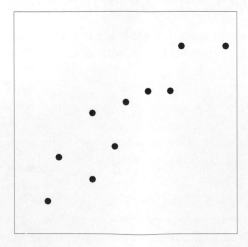

Figure 5.8 'Sample' scatterplot

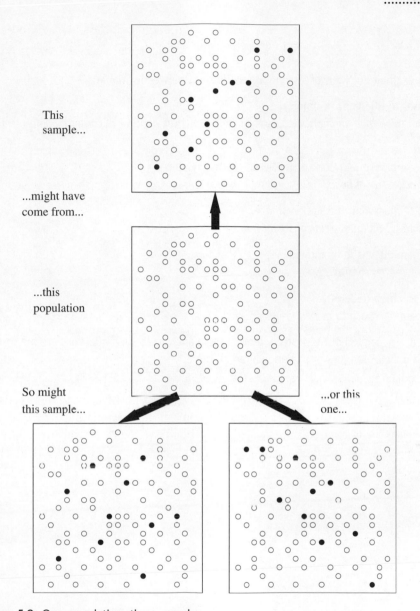

This
sample...

...might have
come from...

...this
population

So might
this sample...

...or this
one...

Figure 5.9 One population, three samples

As in this example, and more generally, the key question in much of the statistical analysis in psychological research boils down to this:

How can the evidence from a sample be evaluated with a view to addressing questions about the population from which the sample came?

Calculations about chance play a central role in trying to get a handle on this problem, and that is why the next chapter is about probability.

CHAPTER REVIEW

This chapter has presented examples of ways of looking at relationships between variables.

- Relating yes/no responses to questions of opinion.
  Example: *Do people who think that criminals should get harsher sentences approve of corporal punishment in school?*

- Relating one variable to another that might plausibly be causally related.
  Example: *Is IQ dependent on size of head?*

- Relating different ways of measuring the same variable.
  Example: *Do two measures of attitudes yield consistent results?*

- Relating subjective judgements made by individuals.
  Example: *Do people rank movies consistently?*

- Relating variables that exhibit a trade-off.
  Example: *Does party-going affect academic performance?*

As in the previous chapter, it was pointed out repeatedly that absolute answers to such questions are not forthcoming from data collected only for samples of the population of interest.

The relevance of probability

IN THIS CHAPTER . . .

. . . relevant ideas about probability are introduced. Why a chapter on probability? The short answer is that the theory of probability is central in allowing researchers to draw conclusions about populations on the basis of data from samples. Accordingly, the necessary groundwork is laid and then straightforward examples are worked through to demonstrate how samples can vary from one to another, and how knowledge of this can allow us to use sample data to make inferences about populations.

MEASURING PROBABILITY

Most people have some conception of probability, even if it's only in connection with gambling or forecasting outcomes of sporting contests. Everyday language includes many terms indicating varying levels of likelihood of something happening which is more or less probable, that is, lying somewhere between impossible and certain – for example, unlikely, improbable, possible, likely, almost certain. Such terms are used routinely in trying to predict events, such as marks in examinations, elections, success in courtship and so on.

What people mean by verbal probabilistic statements is generally vague and subjective. Indeed, research shows that how different individuals interpret a term such as 'probable' varies across a wide spectrum. Similarly, in a court of law, the interpretation of 'beyond a reasonable doubt' varies enormously. The vagueness can, in some circumstances, be replaced by mathematical precision (but this precision should not foster the illusion that probabilistic analysis is cut-and-dried – this is far from being the case).

Although people must have been aware of probability, in some sense, since essentially the start of civilisation through observations from everyday life, and although games of chance have been around in most cultures for millennia, an explicit mathematical treatment of probability is a late development within the history of mathematics. What is recognised widely as the first major contribution came as the result of French gamblers in the seventeenth century appealing to their mathematical friends for practical advice. Such chance procedures as tossing a coin, throwing a die or picking a card at random offer familiar contexts for illustrating how probability can be measured, and this is where we start.

BEFORE READING ON . . .

Try these to see how much you know.
   What is the probability of:

1   Getting heads if you toss a fair coin?

2   Getting 1 head and 1 tail if you toss a fair coin twice?

3   Getting a 6 if you roll a fair die?

4   Getting a score of less than 3 if you roll a fair die?

5   Picking a club, if you pick a card at random from a pack of 52 cards (no jokers)?

6   Picking a card that is *not* an ace, if you pick a card at random from a pack of 52 cards (no jokers)?

7   The first spinner in Figure 6.1 ending up pointing to 1?

8   The second spinner in Figure 6.1 ending up pointing to 1?

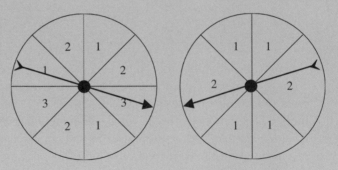

Figure 6.1 Spinning arrows – what is the probability of each arrow finishing on a '1'?

. . . now read on

The answers to the questions follow. If you weren't able to answer most of them with confidence, you may want to brush up on basic probability using an introductory text.

1   The probability of getting heads if you toss a fair coin is $\frac{1}{2}$. In fact, that is what is meant by it being 'fair' – there are equal chances of heads and tails:

$$P(H) = P(T) = \frac{1}{2}$$

where P(H) is convenient notational shorthand for 'the probability of heads' and P(T) for 'the probability of tails'.

2   For the tossing of a coin twice, Figure 6.2 shows two different points of view. Are you convinced by either? Think about it before moving on.

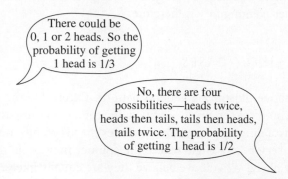

Figure 6.2 Tossing a coin twice – what are the possible outcomes?

The second explanation is the correct one. There are four equally likely outcomes, not three. (The misconception that there are three, as illustrated in the first argument in the figure, is common. If you are not convinced, you could carry out an experiment. Toss a coin twice a large number of times (at least 300) and observe on how many occasions you get one head and one tail (in either order). For a large number of coin tosses, we confidently predict it will be close to $\frac{1}{2}$, rather than $\frac{1}{3}$, of the number of times you did it). Notationally:

$$P(HH) = P(HT) = P(TH) = P(TT) = \frac{1}{4}$$

$$P(1\ \text{head}, 1\ \text{tail}) = P(HT) + P(TH) = \frac{1}{2}$$

where P(HH) means 'probability of heads followed by heads', P(HT) means 'heads followed by tails', and so on.

3   Again, a 'fair' die means that all six numbers are equally likely, so the probability of getting a 6 (or any other particular number) is $\frac{1}{6}$

$$P(1) = P(2) = P(3) = P(4) = P(5) = P(6) = \frac{1}{6}$$

4   A score of less than 3 means either 1 or 2. There are two chances out of six equal chances, so the probability is $\frac{2}{6}$ ($= \frac{1}{3}$).

5   To pick 'randomly' means, by definition, that each card has an equal chance of being picked. Since there are fifty-two cards, of which thirteen are clubs, the probability of picking a club is $\frac{13}{52} = \frac{1}{4}$.

6   There are forty-eight cards that are not aces, so the probability of not picking an ace is $\frac{48}{52} = \frac{12}{13}$.

7   There are eight sectors of equal size, of which three are labelled '1', so the probability of the spinner finishing in one of these is $3/8$.

8   There are six sectors, of which four are labelled '1', *but they are not of equal size* – the sectors labelled '2' are twice as big – so the required probability is *not* $4/6$. In fact, the circle is divided equally into '1' and '2' sectors, and the probability of the spinner pointing to 1 is therefore $1/2$.

EQUALLY LIKELY CASES

The examples above illustrate a general pattern. Except for the final example, where the outcomes as originally defined by the sectors on the spinner are *unequal,* there are a number of possible outcomes (heads or tails, numbers on dice, cards in a pack, sectors of a circle where the spinner may come to rest), each of which is equally likely. Why do we believe they are equally likely? Because there is no reason to believe any one is more likely than any other one. For example, a dice is as perfectly precise a cube as the limitations of manufacture allow, and therefore symmetrical. Similarly, thorough shuffling of a pack of cards means that we have no basis for saying that any one card is more likely to be picked than another.

In these circumstances, if n is the number of possible outcomes ($n = 2$ for a coin, 6 for a standard dice, 52 for picking a card, 8 for the first spinner) then:

the probability of a particular outcome is $1/n$

We may be interested in the probability, not of a single outcome, but of a set of outcomes – for example, what is the probability of getting an even score with a die? Such a set of outcomes is called an *event*. The event 'even score on dice' covers three outcomes – 2, 4, 6. Similarly, for picking a card, the event 'a spade', covers 13 outcomes. If m is the number of outcomes in an event (out of n equally probable outcomes) then:

the probability of the event is m/n

(This includes the special case when the event consists of just a single outcome, in which case the probability is, of course, $1/n$.)

Sometimes we are interested in the probability of an event *not* happening. In that case, if the event corresponds to m outcomes, there are $n - m$ outcomes corresponding to the event not happening, so:

the probability of the event not happening is

$$(n - m)/n = 1 - m/n$$

That is, P(event not happening) = 1 – P(event happening).

Using this definition of probability, all probabilities must lie between 0 and 1 (this should be clear – if it isn't, think about it!). The closer to 1, the higher the probability, the closer to 0, the lower. In the extreme, the probability of an impossible event (such as getting a score of 7 on a normal die) is 0 (since $^0/_n = 0$), and the probability of a certain event (for example, getting a score of less than 7 on a normal die) is 1 (since $^n/_n = 1$).

LONG-RUN FREQUENCY

It is only in special cases that it is reasonable to assume equal likelihoods for the different possible outcomes. Even a coin or die may be biased (that is, have unequal probabilities for different outcomes). A simple example is the following. If a tack is thrown in the air and allowed to fall on the ground, it can land on its back with point straight in the air, or at an angle, with point facing down. Intuitively, we feel that there is a probability for each of those outcomes, but we have no reason to assume that each has the probability $1/_2$. While we cannot determine the probabilities by argument, we can estimate them by experimentation. The tack is thrown many times, and the proportion of times it falls in each of the two positions provides an estimate of the respective probabilities.

In this situation, we can think about the infinite population of possible tosses of the tack. Conceptually, there is a fixed probability, p, for this population, that the tack will land point up (and conversely, a probability $1 - p$ that it will land point down). Any experiment with a number of tosses of the tack provides a sample from this population. From that sample, p can be estimated. Figure 6.3 shows how one such sampling might conceivably go (but of course it will happen differently every time it is done). In the short run, the relative frequency may fluctuate considerably, but in the long run, it can be expected to settle down within a relatively small interval close to the (idealized) true probability.

For this conceptualization of probability to be applicable, it is necessary that:

- essentially the same procedure can be repeated over and over (the technical term for each repetition is **trial**); and

- it is reasonable to postulate that the probability of the event of interest on each trial is independent and constant.

'Independent' means that what happens on any one occasion is not dependent in any way on what happened before.

If these conditions are met, and if the event of interest occurs k times in n replications, its probability, p, can be estimated as k/n. *In general, the larger the number of replications, the better the estimate will be*. It should be clear that a probability estimate derived in this way must lie between 0 and 1.

If the probability of an event is known, or estimated, to be p, then in N independent trials, the event can be expected to happen *about $p \times N$ times*. For example, if a student is postulated to guess every answer in a 40-item multiple choice test with four alternative answers on each item, then the probability of a

Successive sets of 10 trials at a time

N_{up} out of 10	4	2	3	6	5	5	6	7	2	1	4	4	3	3	4	3	5	2	6	3
Total so far	4	6	9	15	20	25	31	38	40	41	45	49	52	55	59	62	67	69	75	78
Percentage so far	40	30	30	38	40	42	44	48	44	41	41	41	40	39	39	39	39	38	39	39

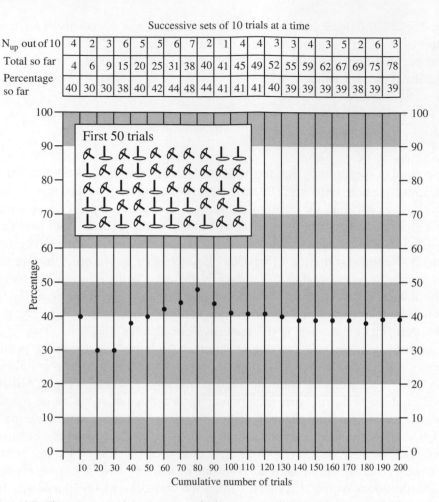

Figure 6.3 Throwing a tack in the air – which way up will it land over 200 trials?

correct choice for each item is $\frac{1}{4}$ and the student would be expected to get *about* 10 (= $\frac{1}{4} \times 40$) answers right 'just by chance'.

SUBJECTIVE PROBABILITY

There are other situations where we feel that we can subjectively make a probabilistic statement, yet there is no basis for doing so, either on grounds of equal probability, or by reference to replications. For example, we may believe that it is almost certain that our team will beat the opposition in a sports event, or that a certain actress will win an Oscar. Such a judgement is called a **subjective probability**, and the person making it could be asked to convert it into a numerical value between 0 and 1. Subjective probabilities play no essential part in this book, however, and are mentioned here only for completeness.

EXAMPLES

As you will see later, in interpreting results of statistical tests, a probability of $1/20$ or less is conventionally taken as meaning 'unlikely' ($1/20$ can alternatively be expressed as a decimal, .05, or as a percentage, 5 per cent). Conversely, a probability of $19/20$ (.95 or 95 per cent) or greater represents a conventional standard for 'likely'. Figure 6.4 presents some examples to give you a feel for what such probabilities mean. In the first example, the probability of picking a black ace (ace of spades or ace of clubs) from a properly shuffled pack of 52 cards is $2/52$, or approximately .038, which is less than .05 ($1/20$). In the second example, with twenty equal sectors on the spinner, the chance of the pointer finishing on the shaded sector is $1/20$. The third example shows the 36 possible outcomes if two dice are thrown. The probability of a total of 12 is $1/36$, = approximately .028, since in only one case is the total 12 (6 and 6). Conversely, the probability of not picking a black ace is approximately .962, the probability of not landing on the shaded

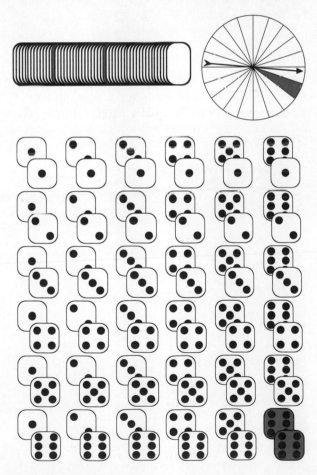

Figure 6.4 'Likely' and 'unlikely' events

sector is $^{19}/_{20}$ or .95, and the probability of getting a total less than 12 is approximately .972.

COUNTING HEADS

As has already been discussed, if a coin is tossed twice, there are four possible outcomes, namely HH, HT, TH, TT. If we are interested in the number of heads (regardless of order) then the probabilities are:

$$P(0 \text{ heads}) = {}^1/_4 \quad P(1 \text{ heads}) = {}^1/_2 \quad P(2 \text{ heads}) = {}^1/_4$$

Now, consider what happens if a coin is tossed four times.

BEFORE READING ON . . .

Can you work out for yourself the probabilities for getting different numbers of heads for four tosses of a fair coin?

. . . now read on

The possible outcomes for four tosses of the coin can be set out systematically as shown in Figure 6.5, and grouped according to the number of heads in each case. Each of the sixteen outcomes is equally likely, with a probability of $^1/_{16}$, so

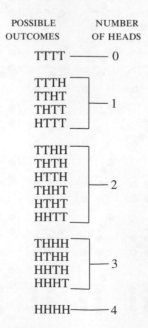

Figure 6.5 Possible outcomes of tossing a coin four times

taking the number of outcomes corresponding to 0, 1, 2, 3, 4 heads into account, the probabilities are as follows:

NUMBER OF HEADS	PROBABILITY	DECIMAL EQUIVALENT
0	$^1/_{16}$	.063
1	$^4/_{16}$	.250
2	$^6/_{16}$	.375
3	$^4/_{16}$	.250
4	$^1/_{16}$	.063

As shown in Figure 6.6, the same information can be presented graphically as a **probability distribution**. Without going into details, the same procedure gives the probability distributions in Figures 6.7 and 6.8 for eight and sixteen tosses of the coins respectively.

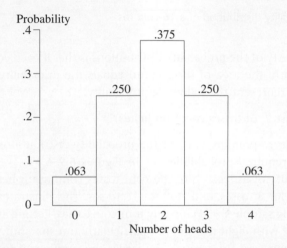

Figure 6.6 Probability distribution of the 4-coin toss

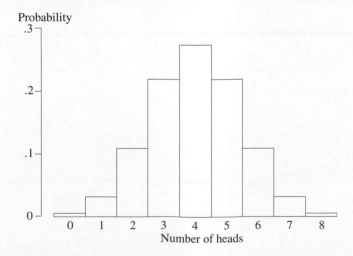

Figure 6.7 Probability distribution of an 8-coin toss

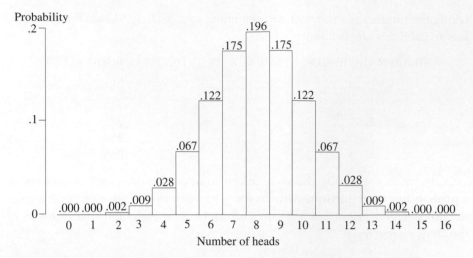

Figure 6.8 Probability distribution of a 16-coin toss

A further property of the probability distributions is that if each column is taken to have unit width, the area of the column equals the probability it represents. Further, we can represent the following probability:

P (at least $^3/_4$ of tosses come up heads)

by shading the corresponding parts of the probability distributions – the shaded areas equal the required probabilities, as in Figures 6.9–6.11. We can then see that the probability of at least $^3/_4$ of the coin tosses coming up heads is .313 for four tosses, .144 for 8 tosses, and .039 for 16 tosses. This illustrates yet again the effect of increasing sample size. With only four coin tosses, getting at least $^3/_4$ heads is quite common, with eight it is still not particularly unusual, but with sixteenth it is less than 5 per cent. In general, the larger the number of tosses, the more likely the proportion of heads is to be close to $^1/_2$.

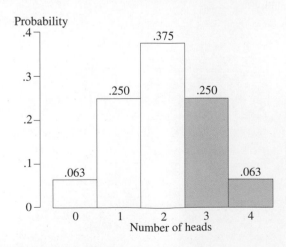

Figure 6.9 Probability of at least 3 heads in a 4-coin toss

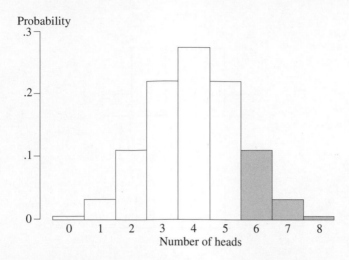

Figure 6.10 Probability of at least 6 heads in an 8-coin toss

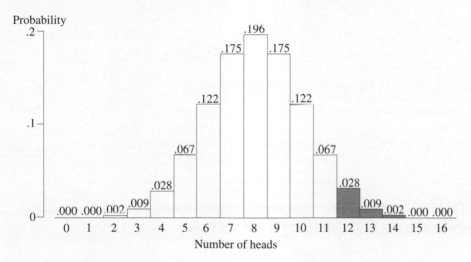

Figure 6.11 Probability of at least 12 heads in a 16-coin toss

THE ROLE OF THE NORMAL DISTRIBUTION

In the examples just considered, the probability distributions have a striking resemblence in shape to the theoretical smooth curve that defines the so-called **normal distribution** (or *Bell Curve*). Indeed, as illustrated in Figure 6.12, the probability distribution for tossing a coin *n* times converges to the *normal* distribution as *n* gets bigger.

As mentioned in Chapter 2, many variables of interest in psychology, when measured for representative samples, produce empirical distributions that reasonably conform to the shape of the *normal* distribution. (It is also important to remember that many other variables produce shapes of distributions which are differ markedly from the *normal* distribution in various respects.)

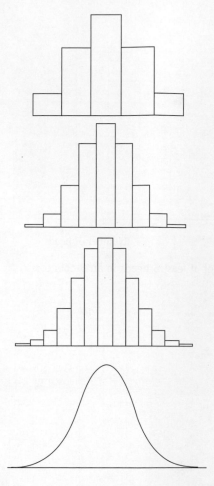

Figure 6.12 Tossing coins – as the number of coins tossed increases, the probability distribution increasingly resembles a normal distribution

The occurrence of roughly *normal* distributions for empirical distributions for variables such as height can be linked to the shapes of distributions presented in the previous section. The number of heads obtained when one tosses a fair coin 16 times may be thought of as arising as the overall result of 16 small causes operating independently, namely the 16 tosses, each of which contributes either 0 or 1 to the total number of heads. The shape of the resultant distribution reflects the fact that there is only one way of obtaining 0 or 16 heads, whereas there are very many ways of obtaining 8. More generally, the number of ways increases towards the middle of the distribution, and falls away to the extremes. A physical characteristic, such as height, could be considered, analogously, as the result of a large number of small causes operating more or less independently – hence the good approximation to the *normal* distribution when height measurements are presented for a sample from a homogeneous population. While this argument is plausible, it should be noted that it is somewhat controversial.

The *normal* distribution is of central importance for another, theoretical, reason. Many of the statistical tests used in psychological research are based on the assumption that the distribution of the variable in question in the population is normal. The technical term for such tests is **parametric** tests. An implication is that, if the distribution of data departs markedly from the *normal* shape, alternative *non-parametric* tests should be considered. This aspect will be discussed at more length in the course of the next two chapters.

PREDICTING AN ELECTION: A SAMPLING EXAMPLE

When an election is taking place, attempts to predict the result on the basis of polls of samples of the electorate are common. Such polls are often badly reported, in the sense that little attention is drawn to sampling variation, although sometimes undefined *margins of error* will be quoted. If one party's estimated share of the vote differs by a few per cent from one week to the next, it is usually analysed on the assumption that there has been a shift in support within the population, whereas the difference may well be attributable to sampling variation; that is, to the fact that the results from different samples of the same population will vary, sometimes considerably.

BEFORE READING ON . . .

Try working through the following exercise that simulates the situation where the voting preferences of a population are being estimated on the basis of a sample. The preferences for three parties – A, B or C – among a population of the electors are represented by the array of letters in Figure 6.13. Obviously, the numbers of As, Bs and Cs in the grid could be ascertained simply by counting. For the purposes of the exercise, however, the whole array of letters will not be counted, only samples. Here's what you should do.

1 Choose a letter, at random, somewhere on the page. Consider the 25 letters forming a 5 × 5 square for which the chosen letter lies at the centre.

2 Count and record the number of As, Bs and Cs in this sample of 25 letters. On the basis of this sample, what percentage of the letters on the entire page would you estimate are As, Bs, Cs? Record your estimate.

3 Now choose another 5 × 5 square (not overlapping the first) and repeat the process. Record the results again. What would your estimates now be for the percentages of letters on the entire page?

4 Repeat the process another eight times, recording the results each time.

Look carefully at all the data you have collected. What do you make of it? Jot down some thoughts.

. . . now read on

Figure 6.13 Electoral preferences (candidates A, B or C) for a population of 2000 voters

Here are the most salient points we would expect you to notice.

■ the percentages of support for parties A, B, and C vary quite a bit over the ten samples;

■ the predicted order of support for the three parties varies from sample to sample, although one party may come out on top more often than the other two; and

- by combining all your samples you get, in effect, a sample of 250. You may have more confidence in the predictions made on the basis of this larger sample.

Now repeat the whole exercise using samples of 49 each time (use a 7×7 square of numbers).

BEFORE READING ON . . .

Look carefully at the data from both parts of the exercise. What differences does a larger sample size make? On the basis of all the information to hand now, how would you estimate the support for the three parties in the population?

. . . now read on

Here are the most salient points we would expect you to notice:

- the variation from sample to sample is almost certain to be less for the samples of 49 than for the samples of 25; and

- with the larger samples, there is a good chance that the indications are that B is the most popular party, followed by A, then C.

If you combined all the samples, you have a total sample of 740 (250 from the first part and 490 from the second). This should give you a fairly good estimate of the actual percentages in the population (which you can find at the end of the chapter).

This example makes a number of absolutely vital points in relation to using samples to make inferences about populations (which is what lies at the heart of standard statistical methods used in psychology):

- a sample should always be interpreted in relation to *what might have happened* with different samples;

- different samples may point to conflicting results (this is really a specific aspect of the first point); and

- the larger the sample, the more stable estimates become, and the more confidence can be placed in them.

A KEY IDEA: CONDITIONAL PROBABILITY

The probability of an event may or may not be changed if we are told that another event has occurred. Examples will make this clearer. If I pick a card at random from a pack (no jokers), the probability that it is an ace is $^4/_{52} = ^1/_{13}$. If I don't look at it, but show it to you and you tell me it's a spade, then, since there are thirteen spades, of which one is the ace, the probability that the card is an ace is still $\frac{1}{13}$. Using notational shorthand:

$$P(\text{ace}/\text{spade}) = P(\text{ace}) = \frac{1}{13}$$

where the first expression means *the probability of picking an ace, given that the card picked is a spade.*

On the other hand, if in the same situation you tell me that the card picked is a court card (jack, queen, king or ace), the probability now that it is an ace is $\frac{4}{16} = \frac{1}{4}$, since the possible outcomes have been narrowed down to sixteen, of which four are aces. In the notational shorthand:

$$P(\text{ace}/\text{court card}) \neq P(\text{Ace})$$

If we reverse the order of the events within the conditional probability, in general we get a different value. For example, the probability of picking a spade given that the card is an ace is $\frac{1}{4}$, since the possible outcomes have been reduced to four (the four aces), of which one is a spade. This is different from the probability of picking an ace given that the card is a spade, which we have already seen is $\frac{1}{13}$.

Similarly, the probability of picking a court card, given that the card is an ace, is 1 (since if it is an ace, it is by definition a court card). Thus:

$$P(\text{court card}/\text{ace}) \neq P(\text{ace}/\text{court card})$$

There are many cases where people get confused about the opposite forms of the conditional probabilities. It may be, for example, that the probability that someone who takes hard drugs previously took soft drugs is high. *It is fallacious to argue from this statement that the probability is high that someone who takes soft drugs will later take hard drugs.* As another example, it is highly probable that a soccer team will win a match, given that they score five goals in the first 15 minutes, but it is *highly improbable* that the team will score five goals in the first 15 minutes, given that they win the match.

BEFORE READING ON . . .

Consider the following information about testing for the HIV virus in a certain population:

- the probability of a positive test result from a person who has the virus = 0.999;

- the probability of a negative result from a person who doesn't have the virus = 0.99; and

- the proportion of people in the population who have the virus = 0.006.

Now suppose a person is diagnosed by the test as HIV positive. What is the probability that the person actually is HIV positive? Make an estimate and record it.

. . . now read on

You may be surprised at the answer. Given the information as stated above, the probability that a person testing positive actually *is* positive is only 0.375, as shown by the following informal proof (it can be proved more formally, but that is beyond the scope of this discussion). Suppose that 1000 people are tested. Then among those 1000 there are about 6 who are HIV positive (given that the proportion in the population is .006). Let us assume that 6 are HIV positive, and the remaining 994 are not. Of the 6 who are HIV positive, the chances are that all 6 will be diagnosed as positive by the test. Of the 994 who are not positive, about 1 per cent will be wrongly diagnosed as positive (see the second piece of information above) – say 10 people – and the other 984 will be correctly diagnosed as negative. Thus, in all, 16 people are diagnosed as positive, of which 6 actually *are* positive and 10 are not. So, if a person is diagnosed as positive, the probability that they in fact *are* positive is only $^6/_{16} = 0.375$ (we repeat, this is not a mathematically impeccable proof, but the same result is obtained by using such a proof). The argument is probably easier to follow through by looking at the diagram in Figure 6.14.

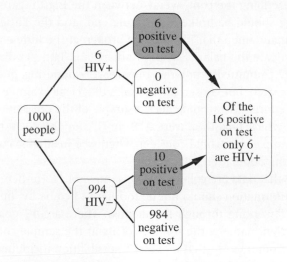

Figure 6.14 What is the probability that someone diagnosed HIV+ *actually is* HIV+?

The chances are that your estimate was much higher. If so, you may have been confusing two conditional probabilities. The probability of a positive diagnosis, given the person has the virus, is 0.999 (as initially stated) – using the notational shorthand:

P(positive diagnosis/person has virus) = 0.999

However, the conditional probability you were asked to estimate was the opposite one – the probability that the person *has* the virus, given a positive diagnosis, and as shown, this is very different:

P(person has virus/positive diagnosis) = 0.375

Confusing one conditional probability with its opposite is very common even among the most educated (and can have serious consequences if used to guide social policy or make decisions, such as in court cases). The reason for analysing this particular example of fallacious probabilistic reasoning is that it is important to be aware of it for a full understanding of the standard method of statistical inference used in psychology, as illustrated in the example that follows.

INFERENCE FROM SAMPLE TO POPULATION: AN EXAMPLE

Having laid some groundwork, we are now in a position to work through a straightforward example that illustrates in detail the logic of standard statistical tests used in psychological research.

In *Gulliver's Travels* by Jonathan Swift, the author satirises political and religious dissension by describing the controversy between the Big-Endians, who asserted that a boiled egg should be broken at the big end, and the Little-Endians, who equally stoutly maintained that it should be broken at the little end. Suppose we wanted to investigate the balance of Big-Endians and Little-Endians in the population at large. (Admittedly not the most earth-shattering question open to psychological research, but chosen for the sake of a clear example to lay bare the logic of the procedure.) We would check a sample of the population and find out for each person which type they were – 'B' or 'L', for short. On the basis of the results for the sample, we would consider whether a justifiable conclusion could be made about the population as a whole.

Let us assume that data are collected for a sample of 16 (rather a small sample, given that the information should not be too hard to come by, but easier to deal with in terms of working through the details). There are 17 possible results of such data collection: namely, the number of Bs in the sample could turn out to be any number from 0 to 16 (that makes 17 possibilities, including 0). If all 16 in the sample turned out to be Bs, that would clearly be pretty strong evidence that there are more Bs than Ls in the population. At the other extreme, if none of the sample turned out to be Bs, that would be strong evidence that there are more Ls than Bs. If the sample turned out to contain 8 Bs and 8 Ls, there would clearly be no indication of an imbalance in the population either way. So far, so obvious. The intermediate cases represent varying degrees of support for Bs or Ls being more prevalent in the population. All of this is summed up graphically in Figure 6.15.

Where do we draw the line? How extreme does the imbalance between the number of Big-Endians and the number of Little-Endians have to be before we consider that the sample offers serious evidence that one group or the other predominates in the population?

To follow one approach to answering this question, we introduce a technical device called the **null hypothesis** at this stage. Before proceeding further,

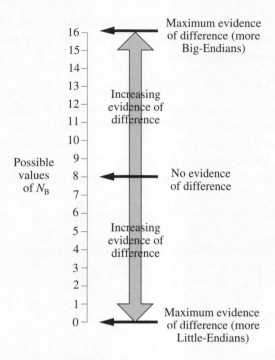

Figure 6.15 Possible numbers of Big-Endians in a sample of 16

however, it is necessary to distinguish two meanings of the word *hypothesis*. Sometimes it is used to indicate something that the speaker believes to be true (but has not yet been proved) as in 'It is my hypothesis that the world is round', or 'It is my hypothesis that English people have a poor sense of humour'. In other circumstances, however, it is a device of formal argument not necessarily believed by the speaker to be true, but taken to be true, literally for the sake of argument. One method of proof in mathematics follows this pattern. For example, the standard proof that the square root of two is irrational (that is, cannot be written as the ratio of two whole numbers) begins by assuming that it is rational and shows how this leads to a contradiction.

In the context of statistical research, the null hypothesis, in general, asserts that no specific effect is in operation (this will become progressively clearer as you encounter more and more examples). For shortness, we use H_0 as notation for the null hypothesis. In the context of the present example, H_0 is that there is no difference either way, that Bs and Ls are equally represented in the population. Here 'hypothesis' is being used in the second sense – for the purposes of following through the argument, it is irrelevant whether or not the experimenter believes it to be true.

The argument now proceeds by asking:

If H_0 is true, what implications follow from that?

Now, we can start to apply some of the probability theory developed earlier. H_0 states that, for each individual in the sample, the probability that they are a B is the same as the probability that they are an L:

$$P(B) = P(L) = \frac{1}{2}$$

We are now in a position to state what the probability is of the sample containing any specific number of Bs if H_0 is true. The situation resembles exactly that already analysed of the tossing of a coin 16 times – each toss of the coin, with a 50/50 chance of heads or tails, corresponds to one person being tested, with a 50/50 chance of being a B or an L (on the assumption that H_0 is true, we repeat). So the probability distribution for N_B, the number of Bs that potentially might be found in a sample of 16, looks like that in Figure 6.16.

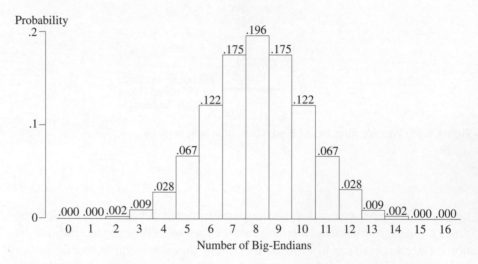

Figure 6.16 Probability distribution for the number of Big-Endians in a sample of 16

N_B is an example of a **statistic**, that is, a number derived from data that reflects some aspect of the data. The probability distribution shown above is called the **sampling distribution** for N_B. From the sampling distribution, we can tell that, if H_0 is true, the probability of N_B taking either of the extreme values is (to three decimal places) .000 (the exact value is $\frac{1}{32768}$). Indeed, the probability of N_B taking a value as extreme as, or more extreme than, 3 or 13, is only .022 (corresponding to the shaded areas in Figure 6.17 and the sum of the corresponding probabilities).

We can thus argue that if H_0 is true, the probability of a result as extreme (in one direction or the other) is very low. We have now reached the pivotal point of the argument. If the experiment is carried out, and the actual result for the sample of 16 is that N_B takes any of the values 0, 1, 2, 3, 13, 14, 15, 16, we consider that doubt has been thrown on the original assumption of the truth of the null hypothesis. The grounds for so doing are that the probability of the statistic taking a value so extreme is very low if H_0 is true.

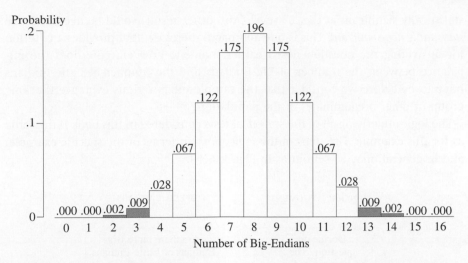

Figure 6.17 Probability that, in a sample of 16, the number of Big-Endians is 3 or less, or 13 or more

If we had included a little more of the tails of the distribution, namely the values 4 and 12, the total probability would have risen to .078, as you can work out from the figure. By convention, a cut-off value of .05 (expressed alternatively as $\frac{1}{20}$ or 5 per cent) is used. If the value of the statistic lies in sections of the tails of the sampling distribution for which the total probability is less than .05, the result is said to be *statistically significant at the .05 level*. Thus, in the present example (illustrated in Figure 6.18), a result for N_B of 0, 1, 2, 3, 13, 14, 15 or 16 would be

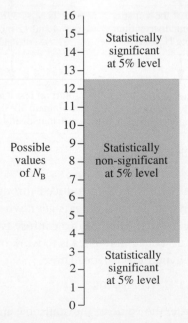

Figure 6.18 Big-Endians and Little-Endians – significant imbalance or not?

statistically significant at the .05 level. Any other result would be deemed to be *statistically non-significant*. This is one approach, therefore, that provides a criterion for answering the question posed earlier, namely: how extreme does the imbalance between the number of Big-Endians and the number of Little-Endians have to be before we consider that the sample offers serious evidence that one group or other predominates in the population?

The logic underlying all of the statistical tests considered in this book is the same as for this example. The steps of the logic, both in terms of the specific example, and in general, may be set out as in Figure 6.19.

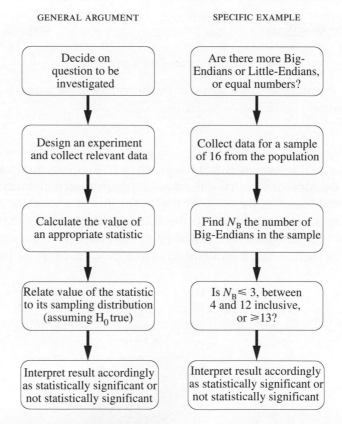

GENERAL ARGUMENT

Decide on question to be investigated

Design an experiment and collect relevant data

Calculate the value of an appropriate statistic

Relate value of the statistic to its sampling distribution (assuming H_0 true)

Interpret result accordingly as statistically significant or not statistically significant

SPECIFIC EXAMPLE

Are there more Big-Endians or Little-Endians, or equal numbers?

Collect data for a sample of 16 from the population

Find N_B the number of Big-Endians in the sample

Is $N_B \leqslant 3$, between 4 and 12 inclusive, or $\geqslant 13$?

Interpret result accordingly as statistically significant or not statistically significant

Figure 6.19 Logic of statistical testing

The notion of statistical significance, introduced through the example, is very easy to misinterpret. Even many statistical texts get it wrong. In particular, people (often quite expert) have a strong tendency to confuse two conditional probabilities. What the approach described here does is to work out statements about the data, given that the null hypothesis is true. Thus:

$$P(N_B \text{ is } \geq 13 \text{ or } \leq 3 / H_0 \text{ true}) = .022$$

In other words, if H_0 is true, the value of the statistic is unlikely to be as extreme as, or more extreme than, 13 or 3. *BUT, the test for statistical significance does not say anything about the probability that the null hypothesis is true, given the data.* For example, if the experiment is carried out and it is found that $N_B = 14$, we have no information from the test for significance about:

$$P(H_0 \text{ true}/N_B = 14)$$

This confusion between the two conditional probabilities is rife and leads, as has been stressed, to major misinterpretations of what is meant by a statistically significant result. It does not give us a handle on the probability that the null hypothesis is true. Instead, a more modest claim can be made. We offer the null hypothesis, as it were, the chance to explain the data. If the data are such that the null hypothesis can offer a plausible explanation, then we give it the benefit of the doubt, or at least we do not reject the possibility that the null hypothesis accounts for the data. However, if the probability of the data given the null hypothesis is low, we look for a different explanation in some systematic effect.

CHAPTER REVIEW

Everyday conceptions of relative likelihood can be converted into precise measures of probability if certain conditions are met. If there are grounds for assuming that outcomes can be assigned equal probabilities, then probabilities of specific events can be calculated. If this is not the case, but the same situation can be replicated over many independent trials, then the probability of an event can be estimated by relative frequency of occurrence in the long run. A crucial point in this regard is that the precision of the estimate is greater, the greater the number of trials.

The normal distribution is important for two main reasons. The first is that the distribution of many variables of interest in psychology at least approximates to its shape. This observation is linked to the second reason, that many statistical tests are based on the assumption that the dependent variable is normally distributed in the population.

You worked through a simulation of what happens when the results of an election are being forecast. From this, certain key characteristics of sampling will have become obvious – in particular, that the results obtained vary, often considerably, from sample to sample, and that more confidence can be placed on larger samples. Since the data for almost all psychological research is collected only for a sample of the population, it is essential to understand these ideas for the interpretation of such research.

An example was worked through in detail to show the basic logic of the method of statistical inference (meaning inference from results from a sample to conclusions about a population) based on the concept of the null hypothesis. This shows how probability is implicated, since the strength of the evidence is gauged by considering the probability of a result as extreme as that obtained occurring if the null hypothesis is true. It was stressed that it is important not to confuse this conditional probability with the opposite conditional probability, namely, the probability of the null hypothesis being true, given the data.

Note: The figures for Figure 6.13 are: 29% of the letters are As; 40% are Bs; and 31% are Cs.

CHAPTER

7 Statistical tests: Comparing

IN THIS
CHAPTER
- - -

. . . we show how the process of testing for statistical significance, introduced through a simple example in the previous chapter (refer back to the figure on page 92 for an overview) is applied to the kinds of question of *comparison* treated graphically in Chapter 4. Specifically, appropriate statistical tests are described for:

■ comparing proportions of participants falling into independent categories;

■ comparing scores between two independent groups; and

■ comparisons based on paired data.

COMPARING PROPORTIONS

The first type of comparison to be considered is for experimental designs in which participants fall into one of several discrete categories (that is, where the variables are *nominal*). The resulting data are in the form of frequencies or proportions. Figure 7.1 presents some data from a sample of students, male and female, concerning whether or not they had used computers before coming to university. Note the totals at the ends of the rows and bottoms of the columns – the overall

	YES	NO	TOTAL
FEMALES	43	60	103
MALES	34	22	56
TOTAL	77	82	159

Figure 7.1 Experience of computers (Yes/No) by gender – frequencies

	YES	NO
FEMALES	41.8%	58.2%
MALES	60.7%	39.3%
TOTAL	48.4%	51.6%

	YES	NO	TOTAL
FEMALES	55.8%	73.2%	64.8%
MALES	44.2%	26.8%	35.2%

Figure 7.2 Row and column percentages

total of 159 students included 103 females and 56 males, and split into 77 who had used a computer before and 82 who had not.

It makes sense to recast these data as percentages, as shown in Figure 7.2. Note that there are two tables of percentages, depending on which way we look at the data (make sure you understand what is going on here). The first table of percentages is more interesting. It shows that while just under half (48 per cent) of the sample had used computers before, proportionately more males (61 per cent) than females (42 per cent) had done so. This imbalance can be shown diagrammatically as in Figure 7.3.

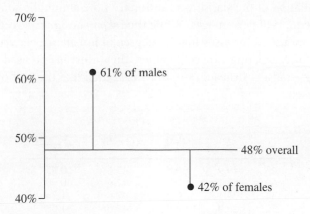

Figure 7.3 Experience of computers – graph of 'Yes' responses showing gender imbalance in relation to overall sample

Is this degree of imbalance indicative of a gender difference in the population from which the sample was drawn, or is it attributable simply to sampling variation? The next step should be clear by now – we need a statistic that reflects the degree of imbalance and which can be related to its sampling distribution.

Again, we state simply that the statistic defined in what follows is an appropriate statistic to use. You will at least be able to see that it does reflect the degree of imbalance between the genders in the sample. To measure the imbalance, we first establish what a balanced situation would look like, and then measure how far the observed data are away from that balance. Given that the overall percentage in the sample was 48 per cent, we calculate what the numbers would look like if the percentage for both males and females were the same, that is, 48

Observed frequencies   'Expected' frequencies

	YES	NO	TOTAL
FEMALES	43	60	103
MALES	34	22	56
TOTAL	77	82	159

	YES	NO	TOTAL
FEMALES	49.9	53.1	103
MALES	27.1	28.9	56
TOTAL	77	82	159

Figure 7.4 Observed and 'expected' frequencies

per cent also. This gives a table of **expected** values that we can set alongside the table of **observed** values, as shown in Figure 7.4. (The term *expected* here can be interpreted as meaning *what would have happened if the overall percentage had applied uniformly across the board*. Another way to think about expected values is as *those values we would expect the data to approximate, assuming the null hypothesis to be true*.)

To measure the discrepancy between these two tabulated sets of figures, the steps in Figure 7.5 are followed to calculate the statistic, which is call **chi-squared** (pronounced 'khy', as in 'kite', 'squared') denoted by χ^2. Before going on to consider the calculation of the statistic, a cautionary note should be sounded regarding data in the form of percentages. While the *column* and *row* percentages shown in Figure 7.2 are useful for assessing the degree of imbalance between males and females, and for calculating expected values, they must *not* be used in the calculation of the χ^2 statistic. Instead, only *raw frequencies*, like those shown in Figure 7.1, may be used.

O	E	$O-E$	$(O-E)^2$	$\dfrac{(O-E)^2}{E}$
43	49.9	−6.9	47.6	0.95
60	53.1	6.9	47.6	0.90
34	27.1	6.9	47.6	1.76
22	28.9	−6.9	47.6	1.68

$$\chi^2 = \sum \frac{(O-E)^2}{E} = 5.31$$

Figure 7.5 Calculation of χ^2

It should be clear to you now that χ^2, because of the way it is defined, cannot be negative. Second, you should be able to see that χ^2 would be zero if, and only if, the observed and expected values were exactly equal – an unusual and implausible situation indicating perfect balance in the sample, and hence no evidence what ever of any imbalance in the population. It should then be clear that the larger the value of χ^2, everything else being equal, the stronger the evidence from the sample of an imbalance in the population. Figure 7.6 sums it up graphically.

The question that remains to be answered is: how far away from 0 does our χ^2 value have to be before we take it seriously? As in Chapter 6 (see page 88), this

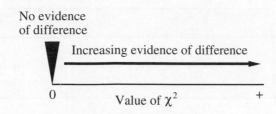

No evidence
of difference

Increasing evidence of difference

0   Value of χ^2 +

Figure 7.6 Value of χ^2 and strength of evidence

is where the device of the null hypothesis proves useful. We begin by assuming there is no imbalance in the population. We then consider the likelihood that our sample data (and resulting χ^2 value) could have occurred, given this assumption. Using the cut-off, or significance, level of .05 discussed in Chapter 6 (see page 91), we identify the threshold, or criterion, value of χ^2 at this level of significance. This is the threshold which our obtained value must equal or exceed to be deemed **statistically significant**. Such threshold values are known as **critical values**, since they are critical in determining whether or not the obtained value of χ^2 is statistically significant. Here we do not attempt to explain any of the technical aspects of how the critical value of χ^2 is derived mathematically. In fact, the value will change with the number of rows and columns in the data table. Suffice it to say that, in the case a 2×2 table, as in our example, the critical value of χ^2 is 3.84 at the conventional cut-off probability of .05 (as discussed on page 91). Since, in the example, the value of χ^2 was found to exceed this critical value, the result is deemed to be *statistically significant*.

A point to which we need to alert you is that, rather than simply confirming whether or not your χ^2 exceeds the critical threshold at .05 level of significance, some statistical software packages give the level of significance as an *exact* probability value associated with the obtained value of χ^2. This is a more precise way of conveying information about statistical significance. If the exact probability value given is .05 (or less), you can conclude that the result is significant.

A further technical point we need to mention is that for the 2×2 case, something called a **correction for continuity** is often applied. This represents a slight change to the formula (which we are not going to detail) for certain mathematical reasons (which we are not going to go into either). We are making the usual assumption about access to software that will incorporate the correction for continuity for you.

A QUESTION OF TASTE

The χ^2 statistic generalises naturally to larger data tables. Figure 7.7 again presents the data introduced in Chapter 4 (see page 46) for preferences among psychology courses, comparing students in two faculties. Overall, 62.9 per cent of the students were in Arts, and 37.1 per cent in Science. If this balance applied uniformly

	PSYCHOLINGUISTICS	SOCIAL	STATS	HCI
ARTS	27	35	3	8
SCIENCE	13	9	3	18

Figure 7.7 Observed frequencies (*Faculty × Favourite Module*)

	PSYCHOLINGUISTICS	SOCIAL	STATS	HCI
ARTS	25.2	27.7	3.8	16.4
SCIENCE	14.8	16.3	2.2	9.6

Figure 7.8 Expected frequencies (*Faculty × Favourite Module*)

to all the courses considered, the 'expected' figures would have been those shown in Figure 7.8.

As in the simpler case above, the χ^2 statistic measures the discrepancy between the eight observed and expected values as follows:

$$\chi^2 = \frac{(27 - 25.2)^2}{25.2} + \frac{(35 - 27.7)^2}{27.7} + \ldots + \frac{(18 - 9.6)^2}{9.6} = 17.52$$

As noted previously, the *critical value* for the statistic depends on the size of the table, since, all other things being equal, the more cells there are in a table, the larger the value of the statistic will be. This is simply because more numbers are involved in the calculation. So, when assessing the significance of our statistic, we need to modulate its value to take account of different sizes of table.

At this point, we need to introduce the term **degrees of freedom** (often abbreviated to **df**). This is a rather technical idea which is seldom well explained in textbooks. We don't propose to add to the confusion in this book. Suffice it to say, in the case of χ^2, df uses the number of rows and columns in the data table to give an indication of its size. In precise terms, df is calculated as follows:

$$df = (r - 1)(c - 1)$$

where *r* is the number of rows (horizontal lines of data) in the table and *c* the number of columns (vertical lines of data). Thus, for a 2 × 2 table, df = 1, and for a 2 × 4 table, df = 3. There are technical reasons why we use the number of rows (and columns) minus 1, but it is not necessary for you to know these. As we shall see, most statistics that we encounter have formulae for calculating associated degrees of freedom.

The following 'mini-table' indicates how the critical value for χ^2 depends on the degrees of freedom:

df	Critical value for χ^2 (at 5% level of significance)
1	3.84
2	5.99
3	7.82
4	9.49
8	15.51
16	26.30

Since, for df = 3, the critical value for χ^2 is 7.82, the value 17.52 of χ^2 for the example is statistically significant.

RED ALERT

It's very easy to abuse the χ^2 test, and computer software will do it for you gladly. The test is only valid when the appropriate conditions apply. These are that the data within the table should be frequencies, and each observation should be independent – that is to say, the total number of cases should be divided among the cells of the table such that each case contributes precisely 1 to precisely one cell, and these observations are made independently. Thus, for the example of course preference just dealt with, each of the 116 students was in one faculty and chose one course as their favourite, so each student contributes 1 to just one cell of the table. Also, it is reasonable to assume that the preferences held by the students are independent.

If, instead, each student had been asked, for each of the courses, whether they liked the course (scored as 1) or not (scored as 0), and the totals had been tabulated, a very similar looking table would have resulted and the data could have been fed into a computer for analysis.

BEFORE READING ON . . .

Why would it not be right to use a χ^2 test on the data just described?

. . . now read on

The χ^2 test would not be appropriate for data collected in the way described, because the observations are not independent. For example, a student might indicate that she liked Psycholinguistics, Statistics, and Human–Computer Interaction. This student would then be contributing 1 to three of the cells of the table, and these contributions are not independent, as they come from the same person. One check to make is that the total of all the cells in the table equals the total number of cases (usually participants) in the experiment.

As mentioned previously, another careless error (occasionally seen in published work) is to apply the statistic to the percentages rather than to the original frequencies. This is plain wrong! What's more, if you think about it logically you should be able to see why.

COMPARISON BETWEEN INDEPENDENT GROUPS

The next type of comparison to be considered is for cases where numerical (that is, at least ordinal) data are collected on some **dependent variable** of interest for two *separate* groups. This type of experimental design is referred to as an **independent groups design**. When such data are collected, the comparison between the two groups can be brought out by comparing averages (means and medians) and measures of spread (standard deviations and semi-interquartile ranges) and by a variety of graphical resources, including multiple line plots, back-to-back stem-and-leaf plots, frequency diagrams, box-and-whisker plots, and a ranking of the combined data (see Chapter 4, pp. 51–2). Now we want to go beyond comparisons based on summary statistics and graphs to introduce a statistic which can be tested for statistical significance following the general procedure introduced in the previous chapter.

At first sight, the obvious candidate for such a statistic, reflecting the difference between the two groups, is simply the *difference between the means*. The following example is designed to show why that won't work.

Consider the two data sets shown in Figure 7.9. For the sake of concreteness, assume that the data are from an experiment on computer attitudes among females. One group of ten females watched a video intended to promote positive attitudes towards computers among females, while a separate group of ten females were not shown the video. (Note: for simplicity, we have used equal group sizes – often, in real experiments of this type, you are likely to end up with unequal numbers.) Computer attitudes were then measured using the questionnaire

Data set A		Data set B	
VIDEO	NO VIDEO	VIDEO	NO VIDEO
73	63	66	52
72	61	62	66
68	57	74	61
66	69	71	77
77	66	85	70
65	71	79	55
70	58	78	59
78	68	82	79
76	60	65	72
75	67	58	49
Mean = 72	Mean = 64	Mean = 72	Mean = 64

Figure 7.9 Computer attitudes – contrasting data sets

described in Chapter 2 (see page 24). Recall that participants can score between 20 (extreme negative score) and 100 (extreme positive score) on this measure.

For the purpose of illustration, let's consider two *possible* outcomes in which the mean score for the *video* treatment is 72, and the mean for the *no video* control treatment is 64, so the difference between means in each case is 8. However, while the average scores might be identical, there is a noticeable contrast between the two data sets which is of crucial significance in this context.

What we hope you noticed is that the scores in data set A show a much smaller spread than those in data set B. In terms of measures of spread, the difference is clear from the summary statistics in Figure 7.10. The contrast is also obvious from the multiple line plots in Figure 7.11.

Data set A			Data set B	
VIDEO	NO VIDEO		VIDEO	NO VIDEO
13	14	Range	27	30
4	4	Semi-interquartile range	7	8.5
4.62	4.88	Standard deviation	9.07	10.45

Figure 7.10 Summary statistics

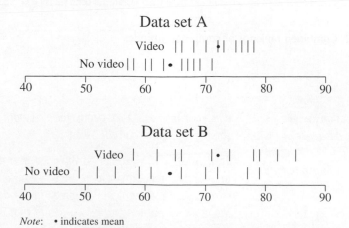

Figure 7.11 Computer attitudes – line plots

BEFORE READING ON . . .

Ask yourself this question: Which data set – A or B – if it were presented to you as the result of the experiment, would make you more likely to conclude that watching the video causes a more positive attitude towards computers among females in general? In considering this question, focus on the data – you can assume that the experiment was well designed and carried out.

. . . now read on

It should be clear intuitively that the answer is 'A'. In data set A, for example, there is relatively little overlap between the *video* and *no video* scores, whereas in data set B there is considerable overlap. (If you think about it, you should be able to see that this is directly related to the much wider spread of scores in data set B.) This can be made even clearer by showing the combined scores for each data set ranked as in Figure 7.12.

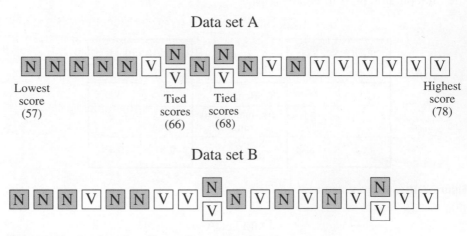

Figure 7.12 Combined rankings of computer attitudes

Statistician: What this demonstration should make clear is the inadequacy of the difference between means as a reflection of the difference between the two groups (video *and* no video *in this example) if we want to reach conclusions about the population in general.*

Student: *I can see that the two data sets have the same difference in means, yet clearly the first data set offers stronger evidence than the second.*

Statistician: *This example is intended also to suggest to you that the extra aspect that needs to be taken into account is the amount of spread in the data within the groups. The standard way of doing that is to use a statistical test called the* **t test**.

THE t TEST

The foregoing argument is by way of introducing the statistic that is normally used in these circumstances, which is called t. You will generally see this referred to in textbooks as **Student's t-test**. 'Is there another test called Lecturer's t-test?' we hear you ask! Actually, the t-test was devised by William Sealy Gossett who worked for the famous Guinness Brewery. As the company did not permit its employees to publish their work, Gossett published his new t-test under the pseudonym of 'Student'. More precisely, since there are other t-tests, the statistical test for comparing two separate groups is called the **independent t-test**, or alternatively, the **independent groups t-test**, or **unpaired t-test** (the last for reasons that will become apparent later). For any two groups in general, which we shall refer to as Group 1 and Group 2 (with means m_1 and m_2 respectively), the formula for t takes the form:

$$t = \frac{m_1 - m_2}{\text{Measure of spread within groups}}$$

Indeed, $m_1 - m_2$ can be thought of as a measure of 'spread' *between* the two groups, making t a measure of spread **between** groups relative to spread **within** groups.

In keeping with the philosophy behind this book, we deliberately do not give the precise formula for the bottom line. If you need to calculate t for a given set of data, we assume you have access to computer software that will do it for you. The technical aspects underlying the derivation of the t statistic lie beyond the scope of this book.

A *simplified approximation* to the precise formula for t is the following:

$$t = \frac{m_1 - m_2}{s_1 + s_2} \times \sqrt{n_1 + n_2}$$

where s_1 and s_2 are the standard deviations for Group 1 and Group 2, respectively, and n_1 and n_2 are the numbers in Groups 1 and 2 respectively. This simplified formula will provide a very good approximation if n_1 and n_2 are equal or roughly equal, and not too small; and if s_1 and s_2 are roughly equal – it's not so good otherwise. The advantage of this simplified approximation to the exact formula is that it shows clearly how t is dependent on the relationship between three aspects of the data, namely:

1.   Difference *between* groups, as measured by $m_1 - m_2$

2.   Variation *within* groups, here approximated by $s_1 + s_2$

3.   Total number of cases, that is, $n_1 + n_2$ (all else being equal, the value of t will double if the number of cases is increased by a factor of 4, for example)

Looking at the formula for t, and bearing in mind that the measure of spread within groups is defined in such a way that it is always positive, you should be able to see that t can be positive, zero, or negative. Clearly t = 0 if and only if the means for the two groups are equal (so that $m_1 - m_2 = 0$), and in this case the sample data would offer no evidence whatever of a difference in the population. When the means are not equal (which in practice will almost always be the case) the value of t is positive or negative depending on which group has the larger mean. Note also that if the contrast is between, say, *video* and *no video* groups, it is arbitrary whether *video* or *no video* is designated as the first group. Of course, you have to remember which way round it is when it comes to interpreting the results.

The larger the value of t (whether positive or negative) the stronger the evidence would be for a difference in the populations in one direction or another. Figure 7.13 sums this up graphically. The by-now-familiar question that remains to be answered is: *How far away from 0 does t have to be before we take it seriously?* This is where the device of the null hypothesis (introduced in Chapter 6) comes in. It will be remembered that, in general, the null hypothesis states that no specific effect is in operation. In the case of the t-test for independent groups, this translates into the statement that *the populations represented by each sample have identical normal distributions,* and that any difference observed in the means is simply a result of the sampling that produced the data.

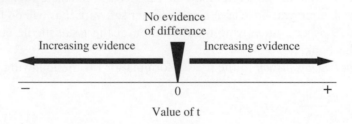

Figure 7.13 Value of t and strength of evidence

Student: I find this idea of samples drawn from populations with identical normal distributions a bit technical and confusing.

Lecturer: In what way?

Student: Well, I can grasp what a phrase like this might mean when you have a subject variable, like gender. There are clearly two populations in such cases.

Lecturer: In your own words, what would be the null hypothesis if gender were an independent variable?

Student: In simple language, the null hypothesis would predict that the average scores on the dependent variable are the same for males and females.

Lecturer: Now, try to use the technical definition to say the same thing.

Student: I would say something like 'the populations represented by the male and female samples have identical normal distributions'. As I said, I'm pretty comfortable with the idea of the entire populations of males and females having the same average scores on a particular measure. But I have real trouble getting my head around what this means in the case of an independent variable that is manipulated.

Lecturer: Ah, OK. I think I see your problem. Let's look again at the previous example [see page 100]. Forget about the technical expression for a moment. In your own words, what is the null hypothesis?

Student: I would tend to express it along the lines of 'there is no overall difference in computer attitudes between the video and no video conditions'.

Lecturer: OK, that's quite specific. Now, try to express the null hypothesis in more general terms.

Student: That's my problem. I find it quite odd to say something like 'the samples represent populations with identical normal distributions' when there is only one

defined population – all females – and both samples are drawn from that population.

Lecturer: This is a good example of the rather arcane language that has grown up around statistics. Here, you have hit on a distinction between the everyday and the technical uses of the term population. In a technical sense, and for the sake of argument, it is perfectly reasonable to think in terms of two populations in this example – the population of females shown the video and the population of females not shown the video.

Student: So, here the population is used in an abstract sense. In my head, this tells me that the video sample is drawn from a theoretical population of all females shown the video. The no video sample represents another theoretical population of all females not shown the video.

Lecturer: It's fine to think of it like that.

HOW DO t-VALUES VARY UNDER THE NULL HYPOTHESIS?

As we have already seen, any two samples drawn from populations with identical *normal* distributions (that is, when the null hypothesis is true) are highly unlikely to have identical means and distributions. They will differ to a greater or lesser extent and, consequently, if we were to calculate the t-value, we would find it to be greater or less than zero. The problem for researchers is that the only data they can evaluate are the sample data themselves. In order to use the t-value to assess the likelihood that the samples represent identical populations, we must have some context. That is, we must know what we might expect if two samples were chosen at random from populations with identical normal distributions, or indeed from a single population.

GETTING A HANDLE ON t

If two samples of 10 are drawn from the same normal distribution, how large might the value of t be? We can use a simulation to get a feel for the answer to this question. For simplicity, the population is reduced to 100 discrete values, arranged so as to give a good approximation to the normal distribution. Two random samples of 10 are taken from this set of 100 values (the same value may be taken more than once) and the value of t for these data worked out.

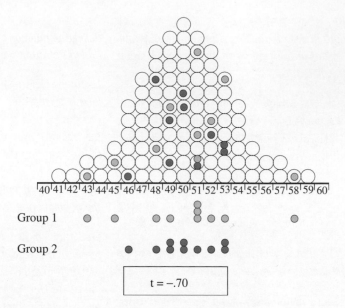

Figure 7.14 Comparing two random samples (*n* = 10)

Figure 7.14 shows one possible outcome of this process, resulting in a value of −.70 for t in this particular case.

If the process is repeated with a different random sampling, the data, and of course the resultant value of t, will be different. By repeating the process a large number of times, a distribution of values of t can be built up. Ideally, we would like you to have access to computer software (or get someone to write it – it's not very complicated) so that you can run the simulation for yourself. If that's not possible, you'll have to make do with results from our running of the simulation. A histogram for 100 runs of the simulation looks like that shown in Figure 7.15. From this diagram, the following important points should be noticed – if t is

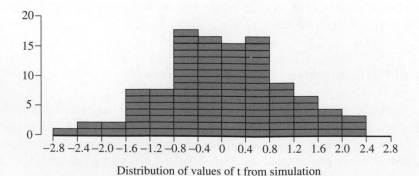

Distribution of values of t from simulation

Figure 7.15 A hundred comparisons of two random samples (*n* = 10)

derived from samples from two populations with the same normal distribution, then:

■ t can be either positive or negative;

■ the values of t for repeated samplings are distributed approximately symmetrically around 0; and

■ values of t beyond ±2 are rare.

As stated, the purpose of introducing this probabilistic simulation is to give you a feel for the distribution of values of t if the null hypothesis is true (the *sampling distribution* for t). In fact, it is not necessary to rely on a simulation, because the exact sampling distribution for t can be derived by mathematical means, the technical details of which lie well beyond the scope of this book. The sampling distribution for t is similar in shape to, but not exactly the same as, that of the normal distribution. It is symmetrical around the value 0. The distribution produced by a simulation is a good approximation to this precise, theoretically derived sampling distribution. A further point is that there is in fact a family of distributions, dependent on the number of cases involved. For a total number of 20 cases, as in this example, the sampling distribution for t is shown in Figure 7.16.

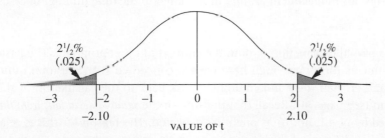

Figure 7.16 Sampling distribution of t (*N* = 20)

Thinking back to the procedure introduced in Chapter 6, we need to specify extreme intervals (called **tails of the distribution**) which correspond to a probability of .05, or 5 per cent. This means, in graphical terms, cutting 2.5 per cent (or .025, expressing it as a decimal) of the area under the curve from each end of the distribution. This amounts to taking the parts of the distribution that lie beyond ±2.10 as indicated in the diagram. What this means is that, for $n_1 + n_2 =$ 20, under the assumption that the null hypothesis is true, the probability of a t value more extreme than ±2.10 is 5 per cent, that is, by the cut-off conventionally used, it can be considered unlikely. Accordingly, if an experiment is done that fulfils these conditions, and the value of t resulting from the data is more extreme than ±2.10, the result is said to be statistically significant at the .05 level; if not, the result is said to be statistically non-significant. Again, the values ±2.10 are called **critical values**, since they are critical in determining whether or not the value of t is statistically significant. Figure 7.17 sums this up graphically.

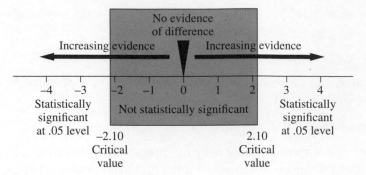

Figure 7.17 Value of t and strength of evidence – critical values and statistical significance

Thus, in practical terms, all that needs to be done is to find the value of the t statistic and check it against the critical value, which depends on the total number of cases, $n_1 + n_2$. Note that, although we have used examples with n_1 and n_2 equal, there is no requirement for them to be equal.

As was the case for χ^2, the t-test has associated *degrees of freedom* (df). In the case of the t-test for independent groups, df is related to the total number of cases thus:

$$df = n_1 + n_2 - 2$$

Again, a partial explanation of df in the context of t is appropriate. The basic logic is the same as for χ^2, although here we are concerned with the total number of scores, rather than rows and columns. Think back to the calculation of standard deviation (see page 34). Recall that the sum of the *squared deviations from the mean* is divided by $N - 1$, not N, as might be expected. The reason for this is related to the fact that the sum of the deviations from the mean is, by virtue of the way in which they are calculated, always 0. That means that only $N - 1$ of the deviations are free to vary, since the last one must be equal to minus the sum of the others (in order to make the total for all N equal to 0). In technical language, $N - 1$ is the *degrees of freedom for standard deviation*.

Now consider the case of data for two independent groups. In calculating the variation within each group, deviations from the mean are used – in fact, the formulae above involve the standard deviations for each of the two groups. For each of the two groups these deviations must, again, of necessity, sum to 0. Hence the number of deviations free to vary within the first group is $n_1 - 1$, and similarly $n_2 - 1$ within the second group. Adding these together, the total degrees of freedom when calculating the total variation within groups is $n_1 + n_2 - 2$.

Tables of critical values are readily accessible, but we don't consider them necessary, as we assume throughout that you have access to software that will calculate the statistic and tell you if it is statistically significant. However, to give you a feel for how critical values vary with degrees of freedom, here is a 'mini-table':

df	Critical value for T (at 5% level of significance)
20	2.09
40	2.02
60	2.00
120	1.98

Note that the critical value varies somewhat for relatively low values of df but soon stabilises (and in fact, it never drops below 1.96, no matter how large df becomes). A rule of thumb is that t must be greater than 2 (or less than −2) to be statistically significant.

Again we need to remind you that in software packages the significance level is often quoted, not simply in terms of <.05 or >.05, but as an exact probability. For example, with $n_1 + n_2 = 20$, a t value of 2.66 has an associated probability (p) value of 0.016 (remember, this is the probability of a result as extreme as, or more extreme than, 2.66 if the null hypothesis is true). The link between the value of t and the corresponding p can be seen in relation to the sampling distribution in Figure 7.18.

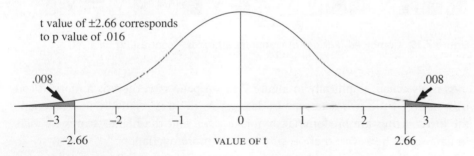

Figure 7.18 Sampling distribution of t ($N = 20$), when t = 2.66, p = .016

Let's return to the two data sets with which we began (see page 100). For the first and second data sets, respectively, the approximate formula for t gives:

$$t = \frac{8}{4.62 + 4.88} \times \sqrt{20} = 3.77 \qquad t = \frac{8}{9.07 + 10.45} \times \sqrt{20} = 1.83$$

You can see how the greater spread within groups in the second data set, reflected in the larger standard deviations, makes the t value much smaller for the second data set. The exact values (to 2 decimal places), as worked out by computer software, are 3.77 and 1.83 (so the approximation works well here) with associated p values of .0014 and .084 respectively. Thus the difference between the groups in data set A, as measured by the t statistic, is statistically significant by a wide margin, whereas the difference between the groups in data set B is not statistically significant by the usual .05 criterion.

MANN–WHITNEY U TEST AS ALTERNATIVE

An alternative statistical test for independent groups is based on ranking the data. Consider the two data sets originally introduced on page 100. For each data set, the combined scores for *video* and *no video* can be ranked, yielding the diagrams shown in Figure 7.19.

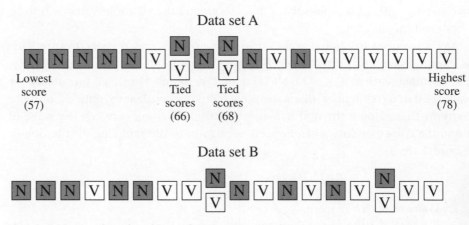

Figure 7.19 Combined rankings of computer attitudes – contrasting data sets

As is also clear graphically in Figure 7.11 on page 101, there is a marked contrast between the two data sets. In data set A, there is relatively little overlap – the lower scores are predominantly for *no video*, and the higher scores for *video*. In data set B, however, there is substantially more overlap.

The U statistic, developed by statisticians Henry Mann and Ransom Whitney, is a measure of the degree of intermingling in the combined rank ordering. One way to define this statistic is as shown in Figure 7.20. Consider the first sequence of Vs and Ns above.

How often in this sequence does a V come before an N? The first V in the sequence comes before 5 Ns, so we count 5 for that. The next V ties with one N (we call that .5) and comes before 4 other Ns, giving a contribution of 4.5 in total. The next V contributes 2.5, and the next 1. The remaining 6 Vs are followed by no Ns in the sequence, so contribute nothing. Adding them all together we get:

$$5 + 4.5 + 2.5 + 1 = 13$$

Repeating the process for the second sequence, we get:

$$7 + 5 + 5 + 4.5 + 3 + 2 + 1 + 0.5 = 28$$

If we do it the other way round, and ask how many times an N comes before a V, we get 87 and 72 as the respective totals. (Note that 13 + 87 = 28 + 72 = 100

Data set A

N N N N N V [N/V] [N/V] N [N/V] N V N V V V V V V

- Comes before 5 Ns in sequence
- Comes before 4 Ns in sequence and ties with 1
- Comes before 2 Ns in sequence and ties with 1
- Comes before 1 N in sequence
- Followed by no Ns in sequence

Figure 7.20 Diagrammatic illustration of Mann–Whitney U

$= n_1 \times n_2$, and this relationship will always hold.) When this process is carried out, the U statistic is the *smaller* of the two numbers obtained – in this case U = 13 for data set A, and U = 28 for data set B.

For 10 Vs and 10 Ns, consider the *possible* sequences. The extreme cases are where there is no overlap at all:

VVVVVVVVVVNNNNNNNNNN

or

NNNNNNNNNNVVVVVVVVVV

and in both cases, U = 0 (think this through, given the definition of U). Thus, a value of U = 0 represents the strongest evidence that one could get from two groups of 10 using the U statistic that there is a difference in the population between the groups. On the other hand, a maximal intermingling of Vs and Ns might look something like this:

VNVNVNVNVNNVNVNVNVNV

giving the greatest possible value U = 50, and representing no evidence whatsoever of a difference between the groups. (In general, the greatest possible value for U is $(n_1 \times n_2)/2$, since U is the larger of two numbers that add up to $n_1 \times n_2$). The closer U is to 0, the stronger the evidence, as is summed up graphically in Figure 7.21.

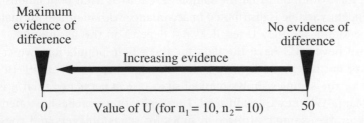

Figure 7.21 Value of U and strength of evidence

The usual question then arises. How close to zero does U need to be to be statistically significant? Here we simply state that the sampling distribution for U for any values of n_1 and n_2 can be worked out (note that n_1 and n_2 don't need to be equal) and the computer will tell you about the statistical significance, or lack of it. For $n_1 = n_2 = 10$, the critical value is 23 (that is, any value of U less than or equal to 23 is statistically significant), so we can augment the diagram as shown in Figure 7.22.

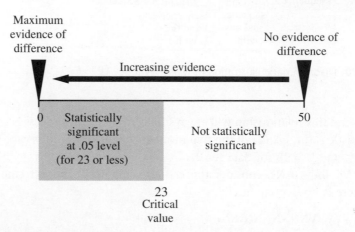

Figure 7.22 Value of U and strength of evidence – critical value and statistical significance

One further technical point needs to be covered. When n_1 and n_2 are large, the U statistic can be converted into a different statistic, z. For the z statistic, the *critical* cut-off value for statistical significance at the p = .05 level is *always* ±1.96, but the software that you use may well give you the precise p that corresponds to your z value.

CHOOSING BETWEEN t AND U

We have said that the Mann–Whitney U test is an alternative to the t-test, but what's the basis for choosing between them? The key point is that the t-test is based on the assumption that the samples are drawn from populations in which the dependent variable is distributed in accordance with identical normal distributions. The Mann–Whitney U test does not depend on this assumption.

Since we never will have the data for the whole population, we cannot tell whether or not it is normally distributed (or a good approximation). However, if the data for the samples shows marked signs of *non-normality*, then it is safer to use the Mann–Whitney U test instead. The implications can be illustrated by referring back to the example of reaction times for squash players and chess players

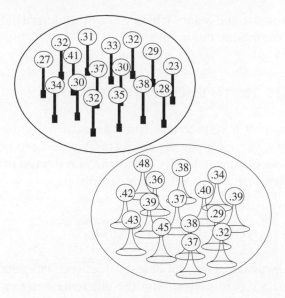

Figure 7.23 *Quick on the draw* – reaction times (sec.) for squash and chess players

analysed in Chapter 4 (see page 50). For convenience, the data are presented again in Figure 7.23.

The distributions of RTs for each group look reasonably like the normal distribution (see graphical representations on page 51, especially Figure 4.12). If we carry out t and U tests for these data the results are as follows:

$$t = 3.87 \qquad\qquad p = .0006$$

$$U = 38.5 \ (z \ \text{equivalent} = -3.229) \qquad p = .0012$$

Consider the effect of adding the two outliers considered previously (see page 52). Recall that the previous difference in RT between squash and chess players disappeared when these outliers were included. Note, though, how the distribution of RTs for the squash players is decidedly non-normal. If we repeat the tests with the amended data, the results are:

$$t = 1.45 \qquad\qquad p = .158$$

$$U = 68.5 \ (z \ \text{equivalent} = -2.409) \qquad p = .016$$

Now the t-test does not produce a statistically significant result, but the U test still does. The U test is much less strongly affected by the addition of the two outliers than is the t-test. The reason for this is that the t-test, because of the way it is defined, is non-resistant (that is, heavily affected by outliers), whereas the Mann–Whitney U test, being based on ranks, is resistant – much less affected by the outliers.

The general rule is, if you have theoretical or empirical reasons for suspecting radical departures from normality in the distribution of the dependent variable, then it is better to use the Mann–Whitney U test. Unfortunately, there are no clear guidelines for making this decision.

COMPARISON WITHIN PAIRED DATA

Recall from Chapter 4 that, in some circumstances, it is possible to make comparisons by testing just one group of participants, but doing so under two conditions – this type of experimental design is known as a **repeated measures design** (since we have repeated measures for each participant).

LET YOUR FINGERS DO THE TALKING

Paralleling our discussion of tests for difference between independent groups, we introduce two data sets to suggest why the difference between means for the two conditions will not work as a statistic for testing for statistical significance. Figure 7.24 shows two data sets which, for the sake of concreteness, represent two possible outcomes for mean typing speed (in words per minute) measured for the same people both before and after a tea-break. In both cases, the mean typing speed before tea-break is 77 and after tea-break 82.

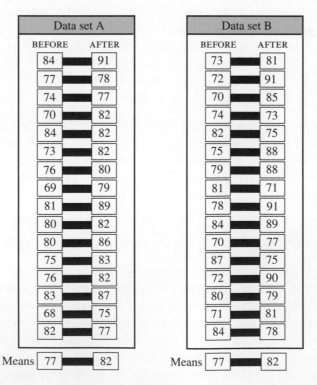

Figure 7.24 Typing speed (wpm) before and after a tea-break – contrasting data sets

Representing the data graphically shows up a marked difference (see Figure 7.25). In data set A, the related line chart shows a consistent increase in typing speed after the teabreak, with only two exceptions to the pattern. In data set B, the results are more mixed in this respect.

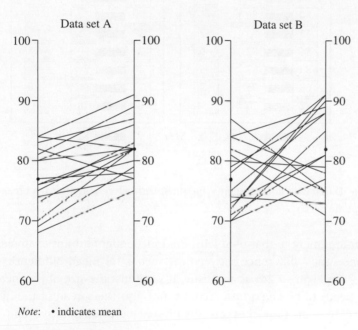

Note: • indicates mean

Figure 7.25 Contrasting related line charts

Further insight can be gained by adding columns to the data to show the before–after differences, as in Figure 7.26. In each case the *after* measure is subtracted from the *before* measure (leading to positive or negative results, depending on which is the larger). The mean difference (m_d), as you can see, is −5 in both cases. What becomes clear from looking at the differences is that they are much more widely spread for the second data set than for the first. This can be measured, for example, by working out the standard deviation for the difference (s_d) in each case.

If you think about it, you'll see that this is not unconnected to the contrast already mentioned – 14 out of 16 in data set A showing improved performance after the tea-break, as opposed to 10 out of 16 in data set B.

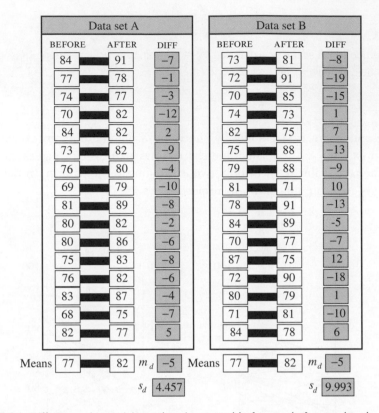

Figure 7.26 Differences in participants' typing speed before and after tea-break – contrasting data sets

A similar argument to that used with the independent groups example leads us to reject the simple difference between the means (or mean difference, which is the same – see Figure 7.26) as a statistic. It's not just the size of the mean difference that needs to be taken into account, but also the spread of the differences and, linked to that, how they are distributed between positive and negative values.

t-TEST FOR PAIRED DATA

The argument presented above is by way of introducing the standard statistic for comparisons between paired data sets. It is called the **paired t-test** (or **correlated t-test**) and the formula is:

$$t = \frac{m_d}{s_d} \times \sqrt{N}$$

The reason why it is also called t is that it has the same sampling distribution as the independent t-test. (Subscripts can be used, if necessary, to differentiate the two uses of the statistic, t_{ind} for independent groups t-test, and t_{paired} for paired t-test).

The formula takes into consideration not only the mean difference but also the spread of the differences as measured by the standard deviation and, furthermore, the number of pairs (N). The degrees of freedom for the paired t-test is 1 less than the number of pairs, namely $N - 1$. Analogously to the formula for degrees of freedom for the independent t-test, the formula $N - 1$ reflects the fact that, in calculating the standard deviation of the differences, only $N - 1$ of the deviations from the mean are free to vary.

Otherwise, the criterion for significance or non-significance (or *critical* t value) is similar to that used in the case of the independent t-test. Again, a rough rule of thumb is that the value of t must be more extreme than ±2 to be significant (the precise critical value varies with N (and hence df) as indicated in the 'mini-table' on page 109).

For the data sets used in the example, the values of t are:

$$t = \frac{-5}{4.457} \times \sqrt{16} = -4.49 \qquad t = \frac{-5}{9.993} \times \sqrt{16} = -2.00$$

The critical value is 2.13 for $N = 16$ (df = 15). Thus, you can see that for data set A, the difference is clearly statistically significant, whereas for data set B, it is not.

SIGN TEST AS A SIMPLE ALTERNATIVE

There is a very simple alternative test for paired data. It is based on counting the number of pairs for which the first score is higher, and the number for which the second score is higher (if there are any ties, they are ignored). For data set A in the example there are two cases where the before tea-break performance is better, and fourteen where the after tea-break performance is better. The corresponding figures for data set B are six and ten.

In fact, the sampling distribution for this statistic has been discussed already in Chapter 6 (see Fig.6.8 on page 80). The null hypothesis for the sign test is that, for each individual, the difference is as likely to go one way as the other. The situation, therefore, is exactly analogous to tossing sixteen coins and counting the number of heads. It was shown in Chapter 6 that an imbalance in this situation as great as 13:3 in either direction represents a statistically significant result, but any lesser imbalance is not statistically significant. Hence, by the sign test, data set A yields a statistically significant result, whereas data set B does not.

For larger N, the statistic can be converted to a value of z, which can then be compared with the critical value ±1.96 (as with the Mann–Whitney U test). Again we assume that the software you use will do this. For this particular example, the sign test is not a particularly good choice, and either t_{paired} or the rank-based test we are about to deal with is better.

ANOTHER ALTERNATIVE – THE WILCOXON MATCHED PAIRS SIGNED RANKS TEST

Just as the Mann–Whitney U test is a rank-based alternative to t_{ind}, the Wilcoxon Matched Pairs test (yes, devised by Frank Wilcoxon) is a rank-based alternative to t_{paired}. To see how it works, look again at the illustrative data sets, with the differences calculated.

Whereas the sign test merely takes into account whether the differences are positive or negative, the Wilcoxon Matched Pairs test also takes into account the size of the differences. This is done by ignoring the sign initially and ordering all the differences. Figure 7.27 shows the result for data set A. The statistic for this test, denoted by W, is the sum of the ranks associated with the less frequent sign (in this case positive). For data set A, W = 9.5, as shown.

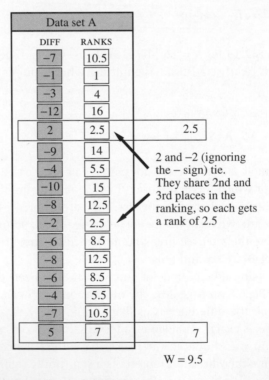

Figure 7.27 Calculating Wilcoxon's W

BEFORE READING ON . . .

To check that you follow the procedure correctly, calculate W for data set B.

. . . now read on

It should be clear that W will equal zero if, *and only if,* all the differences are in one direction (positive or negative). This would constitute the strongest evidence on the basis of this test for a difference between the two conditions. Due to the way it is defined, W is by nature non-negative. The larger it is, the less strong the evidence of a difference in the population between the scores for the two conditions.

Again, the critical values for small N can be calculated exactly, while for large N, the value of W can be converted into a value of z to test for statistical significance.

In the case of our example, with $N = 16$, the critical value is 14. Hence, as you might expect, data set A yields a statistically significant result, while data set B (you should have calculated W to be 33) does not.

CHOOSING BETWEEN t_{PAIRED} AND WILCOXON

As with the tests for comparing independent groups, the choice of tests for paired data hinges on the conditions necessary for the test to be appropriate. t_{paired} is based on the assumption that the differences between the paired scores are normally distributed in the population. If there is indication from the data that this assumption is not reasonable, the Wilcoxon is a more careful choice to make. As with the previous contrast between t_{ind} and Mann–Whitney U, t_{paired} is a less resistant test than the Wilcoxon. But again there are no clear guidelines for making the choice.

ANOTHER CASE OF PAIRED DATA: MATCHED PAIRS DESIGNS

For the repeated measures design we have been discussing, the data are paired by virtue of the fact that each pair is linked to a single individual. Here we consider another type of experimental design – the **matched pairs design** – that results in paired data for a different reason, which we illustrate with an example.

BOYS' AND GIRLS' MATHEMATICAL ABILITIES

Suppose a researcher wished to test whether 9-year-old boys and girls differ in mathematical ability as measured by some test. Data bearing on this question could be collected by measuring samples of 9-year-olds and comparing their scores using an independent groups t-test. However, the researcher may be worried that mathematical ability is highly related to intelligence, and that the samples of boys and girls might differ in this respect, thus complicating the interpretation of any difference that might be found between the scores for the two groups. One way

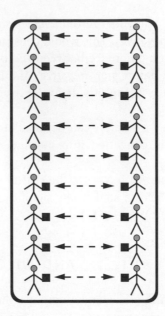

Figure 7.28 Matched pairs design

to avoid this possibility is to test initial samples of boys and girls for intelligence and then, from these samples, choose **matched pairs**; that is, boy–girl pairs of the same, or very similar, measured intelligence. The resulting data could then be analysed using a paired t-test – paired, because the data are paired by virtue of the matching process. A matched pairs design may be represented schematically, as in Figure 7.28.

CHAPTER REVIEW

In this chapter, the general procedure for carrying out statistical tests based on the null hypothesis and testing for statistical significance has been worked through for a number of common experimental designs and corresponding data concerned with comparisons. Specifically, tests have been introduced for:

■ Comparing proportions of responses from different groups.
  Example: *Do the proportions of students preferring various courses differ between two faculties?*

■ Comparing two groups' measurements on some variable.
  Example: *Are attitudes towards computers more positive in a group of females shown a promotional video, compared to a group not shown the video?*

■ Comparing performances of one group of people under different conditions.
  Example: *Do people type more efficiently after a tea-break than before?*

For independent groups and paired data comparisons, more resistant rank-based alternatives to t_{ind} and t_{paired} tests were described.

Statistical tests: Correlating

. . . the workings of more statistics are explained. Whereas the last chapter was about tests for making *comparisons* between two sets of data for different groups of people or paired measurements for a single group of people, this chapter deals with ways of measuring the strength of *relationships* between variables. These methods extend the descriptive analyses of relationships between variables introduced in Chapter 5.

QUANTIFYING STRENGTH OF RELATIONSHIP

In Chapter 5, the use of scattergrams to illustrate the relationship between pairs of variables was illustrated by several examples. Further, it was shown how an initial rough idea of the nature of the relationship could be obtained by dividing the scattergram into quadrants by vertical and horizontal lines through the mean value for the respective variables.

As a reminder, three of the examples are reproduced in Figure 8.1. The first shows the relationship between height and weight for a sample of sixty male psychology students. The majority of points lie in the A and C quadrants, reflecting a **positive correlation**; that is, (as you would expect) the general pattern is that the taller people are, the heavier they are. The second example shows the relationship between head size and measured IQ. In this case, the points are distributed relatively evenly among the four quadrants, reflecting no strong relationship (where brains are concerned, size is not everything, according to these data). The third example (a work of fiction) shows the relationship between number of parties attended and exam performance. Here the majority of points lie in the B and D quadrants, reflecting a pattern whereby (in general, with some exceptions) the more parties attended, the less good the exam performance, and vice versa. Such a pattern is called a **negative correlation**.

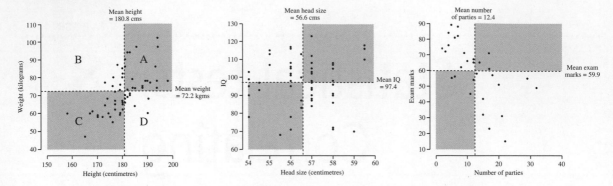

Figure 8.1 Scatterplots – weight/height, IQ/head size, and exam mark/number of parties

ASSIGNING A NUMERICAL MEASURE TO CORRELATION

Now we take the quadrant analysis a step further to introduce a single number which – in a very *specific* sense, to be defined – measures the strength of the relationship between two variables for which data have been collected for a group of participants. A number of this sort is called a **correlation coefficient**. A simpler example with just ten points is used to introduce the formula and work through the calculation.

The formula for this correlation coefficient, the conventional symbol for which is r, is as follows:

$$r = \frac{\sum (X - \overline{X})(Y - \overline{Y})}{\sqrt{\sum (X - \overline{X})^2 \sum (Y - \overline{Y})^2}}$$

While you may consider that this looks complex, it is easy enough to interpret when you know how. Concentrate for now on the top line:

$$\sum (X - \overline{X})(Y - \overline{Y})$$

The capital Greek letter sigma, Σ, indicates summation (that is, adding up). The symbolic expression as a whole tells you to work out $(X - \overline{X})(Y - \overline{Y})$ for each point, and add all the results together. $X - \overline{X}$ is the value of X, for any individual, relative to the mean of all the X values. It can be positive or negative, depending on whether the X value is, respectively, greater or less than the mean. For example, if you got 65 in a statistics test and the mean for the class was 57, then you would have scored 8 above the mean ($65 - 57 = 8$). If you got 53, that would be 4 below the mean, which can be symbolised as -4 (since $53 - 57 = -4$). Similarly, $Y - \overline{Y}$ means the value of Y, for any individual, relative to the mean value of Y for all cases. The technical terms for either $X - \overline{X}$ or $Y - \overline{Y}$ is **deviation from the mean**. The calculation of the top line can be carried out systematically, as indicated in Figure 8.2.

These are the steps in the calculation:

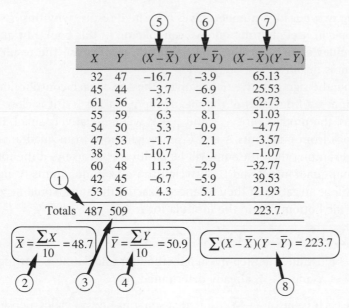

Figure 8.2 Calculation of top line of formula for r

1 Add the *X* values together – the sum comes to 487.

2 Dividing by 10 gives $\overline{X}$ = 48.7.

3 Add the *Y* values together – the sum comes to 509.

4 Dividing by 10 gives $\overline{Y}$ = 50.9.

5 Calculate $X - \overline{X}$ for each case; some are positive, some are negative.

6 Calculate $Y - \overline{Y}$ for each case; some are positive, some are negative.

7 Multiply each value of $X - \overline{X}$ by the corresponding $Y - \overline{Y}$.

8 Add the values of $(X - \overline{X})(Y - \overline{Y})$ together, which comes to 223.7.

BEFORE READING ON . . .

What relationship can you see between the quadrant a point is in and the corresponding values of $(X - \overline{X})$ and $(Y - \overline{Y})$?

. . . now read on

What we hope you have noticed is that points in quadrants A and C contribute positively to the sum, while points in quadrants B and D contribute negatively. In the case of quadrant A, both deviations from the mean are positive – points in this quadrant represent individuals above the respective means for both variables. In quadrant C are individuals with two negative deviations from the mean –

multiplying two negative numbers gives a positive result (why this is so is a fascinating topic in itself, but not one we can take on in this book). In quadrants B and D, one deviation is positive and the other negative, so the result of multiplying them is negative.

Apart from the sign (positive or negative), the size of each contribution depends on how far away from each of the means the point lies – if it is close to one or both means, the product of $X - \overline{X}$ and $Y - \overline{Y}$ will be relatively small. If the total contributions from quadrants A and C outweigh those from quadrants B and D (as in this example) then the sum will be positive; conversely, if the total contributions from quadrants B and D outweigh those from quadrants A and C, then the sum will be negative. If they balanced exactly, the sum would be zero.

Now for the bottom line in the formula for r:

$$\sqrt{\sum(X - \overline{X})^2 \sum(Y - \overline{Y})^2}$$

Figure 8.3 illustrates the step-by-step method for calculating r, starting from the values of $X - \overline{X}$ and $Y - \overline{Y}$ already determined:

1 Square each value of $X - \overline{X}$. (Note that squaring always yields a positive result, regardless of whether the number squared is positive or negative.)

2 Add the results together to get 820.10.

3 Square each value of $Y - \overline{Y}$.

4 Add the results together to get 228.90.

5 Multiply $\Sigma(X - \overline{X})^2$ and $\Sigma(Y - \overline{Y})^2$.

6 Take the square root (positive) of the answer.

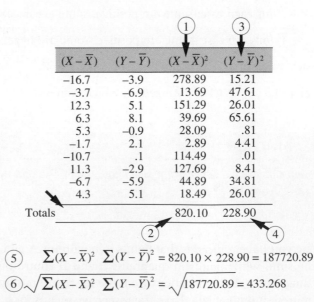

Figure 8.3 Calculation of bottom line of formula for r

We can now find r:

$$= \frac{\sum (X - \overline{X})(Y - \overline{Y})}{\sqrt{\sum (X - \overline{X})^2 \sum (Y - \overline{Y})^2}} = \frac{223.7}{433.268} = .516$$

The bottom line of the formula accomplishes a couple of useful things: (i) because of the way the mathematics works out, it acts as a kind of scaling factor, so that r is forced to lie between −1 and +1 (of which more in a minute); and (ii) It means that r is not changed by changes of the units used to measure the variables. For example, in the relationship between height and weight, if height was measured in inches instead of centimetres, and weight in pounds instead of kilograms, the value of r would not be changed. Since r is intended to be a measure of the strength of the relationship between height and weight, it should be clear intuitively that keeping the same value in these circumstances is a desirable property.

As just mentioned, because of the way it is defined, r is constrained to lie between −1 and +1. In extreme cases, r = ±1 if, *and only if*, the points in the scattergram lie exactly on a straight line (+1 for a perfect positive relationship, −1 for a perfect negative relationship). For real data, it's virtually certain that this degree of exact relationship will never occur, but a more or less good approximation to it will be found when variables are correlated. In general, r may be thought of *specifically* as a measure of 'straightline-ness' (linearity, to use a more technical term). The closer the points in a scattergram approximate to a straight line, the closer r will be to +1 (positive correlation) or −1 (negative correlation).

BEFORE READING ON . . .

To check that you have followed the procedure correctly, calculate r for these data. Just five points have been used to keep the work down for you.

X	7	12	5	14	8
Y	11	9	6	15	10

. . . now read on

You can check at the end of this section whether you got the right answer. A couple of comments are in order as to why, in this case, we have worked through the steps of the calculation in detail, whereas in general we use computer software, making calculation unnecessary. One reason is that the calculations, in this case, should help to give you insight into the way the formula fits together to do the job required. Another is to give at least one example where you can check the answer on the computer and see for yourself that the formula leads to the same result − just to show that the computer is not some black box, but offers a way of carrying out a sequence of well-defined arithmetical procedures.

Statistician: *If there is no general relationship in the data, as in the example of head size and IQ, then the value of r will be close to zero.*

Student: *So a value of r close to zero means no relationship?*

Statistician: *No! I didn't say that. No relationship means r close to zero, but not vice versa. Consider the data in Figure 8.4, for which a scattergram is shown and for which r = zero, to two decimal places. Would you say that there is no relationship between variables X and Y?*

Student: *As X increases, Y does at first but after a certain point it starts to decrease. There's a clear relationship. So why is the value of r close to zero if it is supposed to measure how close a relationship there is between X and Y?*

Statistician: *The point is that r measures 'straightlineness', remember. For these data, there is a relationship, but it's a curved one, not a straight line one: r just isn't capable of detecting this pattern – it's only sensitive to how close the data come to a straight line.*

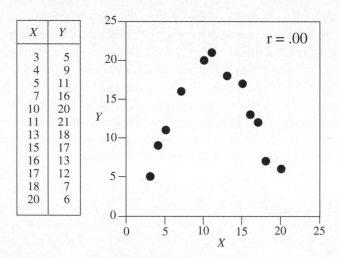

X	Y
3	5
4	9
5	11
7	16
10	20
11	21
13	18
15	17
16	13
17	12
18	7
20	6

r = .00

Figure 8.4 Example of r = 0 – no relationship?

The full title of r is the *Pearson Product-Moment Correlation Coefficient*. It was devised, as you might guess, by a statistician called Pearson (Karl). 'Product-moment' is merely a technical way of describing the way in which the multiplication of $X - \overline{X}$ and $Y - \overline{Y}$ is used in its calculation.

Answer to calculation of r:
r = .74

A RANK-BASED ALTERNATIVE

The Product-Moment Correlation Coefficient is just one of many alternative measures of correlation. Each reflects a different way of looking at the strength of a correlation, is used in different circumstances, and has different characteristics. For our purposes, we need to consider just one more correlation coefficient, the calculation of which is based on ranking procedures.

CRITICAL THINKING

Figure 8.5 again presents the data from Chapter 5 for three critics' rankings of ten classic films (see page 66). A scattergram shows that the judgements of A and B are relatively close, but how can the degree of closeness be expressed numerically? One measure is called the **Spearman Rank-Order Correlation Coefficient** (yes, named after Spearman (Charles)) conventionally symbolised by ρ (the Greek equivalent of r, and pronounced 'roe'). Figure 8.6 illustrates the steps in calculating ρ:

	A	B	C
Battleship Potemkin	6	5	9
Bicycle Thieves	5	3	6
The Birds	10	9	2
Casablanca	9	8	1
Citizen Kane	4	6	5
High Noon	8	10	7
If...	7	7	4
Jules et Jim	2	4	8
Pulp Fiction	3	1	3
Seven Samurai	1	2	10

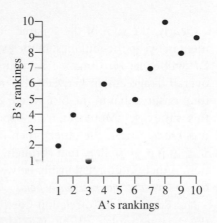

Figure 8.5 Classic film rankings and scatterplot for A/B

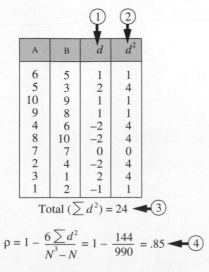

A	B	d ①	d^2 ②
6	5	1	1
5	3	2	4
10	9	1	1
9	8	1	1
4	6	−2	4
8	10	−2	4
7	7	0	0
2	4	−2	4
3	1	2	4
1	2	−1	1

Total $(\sum d^2) = 24$ ◄③

$$\rho = 1 - \frac{6 \sum d^2}{N^3 - N} = 1 - \frac{144}{990} = .85 \quad ◄④$$

Figure 8.6 Calculating ρ

1   Subtract the second rank from the first rank in each case to find the difference, d.

2   Square these differences.

3   Add the squared differences, which comes to 24.

4   Calculate ρ using the formula shown (where N is the number of cases – ten in this example).

BEFORE READING ON . . .

To check that you have followed the procedure correctly, calculate ρ for the rankings of A and C. (You can check your answer at the end of this section.)

. . . now read on

Clearly, the sum of the squared differences reflects the overall level of agreement between the rankings. In the extreme case where the rankings agree exactly, Σd^2 will equal zero (make sure you understand why this is so). The greater the overall disagreement between the rankings, the larger Σd^2 will be. The formula for ρ ensures that in the case where $\Sigma d^2 = 0$, $\rho = 1$ (again, make sure you see why this is the case). Moreover, if the opposite extreme occurs (that is, one set of rankings *exactly reverses* the other), then (as some algebra will show) $\Sigma d^2 = (N^3 - N)/3$ so that $\rho = -1$ (follow that through, too). As with the Product-Moment correlation, if there is no relationship between the rankings, ρ will be close to zero – *but the converse does not necessarily hold.*

The Rank-Order Correlation Coefficient can be used with any variables where the data are ranked. If the original data are measurements on some scale, they can be converted to ranks first, and the same steps as shown above can then be applied to calculate ρ. For example, for the data on page 126, the original 'raw' data for X and Y and the corresponding ranks are as shown in Figure 8.7 (ranking

X	Y	Rank X	Rank Y
3	5	1	1
4	9	2	4
5	11	3	5
7	16	4	8
10	20	5	11
11	21	6	12
13	18	7	10
15	17	8	9
16	13	9	7
17	12	10	6
18	7	11	3
20	6	12	2

Figure 8.7 Data for r = 0 – ranked

has been done here from lowest to highest, but highest to lowest would do equally well, as long as the choice is the same for both variables).

The value of ρ for these data is −.01, to 2 decimal places (you might like to check that by doing the calculations for yourself), illustrating the point that a value of ρ close to zero does not signal automatically the lack of a relationship between the variables. What ρ measures specifically is agreement between rankings, so it is not alert to the U-shaped relationship that is obvious to the naked eye when the data are scattergrammed.

Answer to calculation of ρ:
ρ = −.61

COMPARING r AND ρ

As was emphasised above, r and ρ measure somewhat different aspects of correlation that will not always lead to similar values for the correlation coefficients. To illustrate this, consider the three data sets in Figure 8.8. The summary statistics for all three are the same. However, when the scatterplots are drawn (Figure 8.9), striking differences become obvious. Data set 1 shows a strong linear relationship with the points scattered reasonably close to a straight line, while data set 2 shows an even stronger linear relationship for all the points – with one exception that doesn't conform to the trend of the rest. As we saw before, such an anomalous point is called an *outlier*. Data set 3 is even more strikingly different. Here all the points except the outlier show a negative relationship, and the outlier is very far away. Yet the Product-Moment correlation for all the data sets is .76 – how can this be?

Data set 1		Data set 2		Data set 3	
X	Y	X	Y	X	Y
5	5	5	7	8	11
7	4	7	6	9	10
8	9	8	7	10	12
9	6	9	8	10	9
11	14	11	10	11	13
12	18	12	10	11	10
14	9	14	12	12	9
15	10	15	11	13	14
17	14	17	26	13	11
18	19	18	14	15	7
19	20	19	16	16	8
20	14	20	15	27	28

Mean	12.9	11.8	12.9	11.8	12.9	11.8
s.d.	5.0	5.5	5.0	5.5	5.0	5.5
r		.76		.76		.76

Figure 8.8 Data sets with identical summary statistics

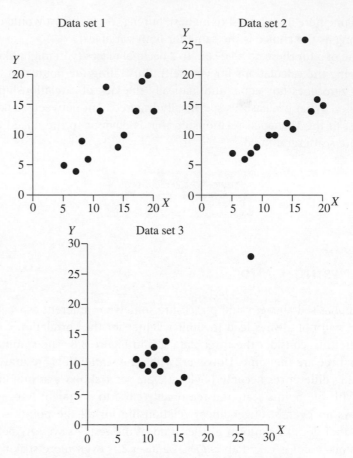

Figure 8.9 Scatterplots of data sets with identical summary statistics

The Product-moment correlation of .76 for data set 1 is clear enough, reflecting the strong linear relationship apparent in the scattergram. For data set 2, the correlation would be much higher than .76 were it not for the effect of the outlier. In the case of data set 3, the outlier dominates the calculation of r, raising it to .76. Here there is in fact a negative correlation between the rest of the points when the outlier is removed.

This example shows how important it is not to rely on summary statistics alone when analysing data. In former times, when computer packages tended to be limited to print-outs giving numerical values of summary and inferential statistics, it was easily possible to misinterpret data by relying only on these statistics. With advances in computer software for personal computers, however, there is no longer any excuse for not taking the time to examine the data graphically, since a package of any quality will make this possible in a matter of seconds. In particular, we would suggest as a general rule: *Never calculate a correlation coefficient without plotting a scattergram.*

Now consider the Rank-Order Correlation coefficients for the same three data sets. For data set 1, $\rho = .79$, close to the value for r. For 'well-behaved' data such as these, r and ρ will, in general, yield fairly similar values.

BEFORE READING ON . . .

Make an guesstimate of the Rank-Order correlation coefficients for data sets 2 and 3.

. . . now read on

The Rank-Order correlation coefficient, ρ, for data set 2 is .93, much higher than the corresponding r. The damping effect of the outlier on the overall outcome is limited. Thus, the Rank-Order correlation coefficient, like other statistics based on ranking procedures, is resistant (that is, not overly affected by outliers); the Product-Moment correlation coefficient, as has been demonstrated, is non-resistant.

The Rank-Order correlation coefficient for data set 3 is $-.01$ (compare this with .76!). Again, the ranking process yields a statistic resistant to the distortion of the outlier. For both data set 2 and data set 3, the Rank-Order correlation coefficient better summarises the overall pattern, not allowing the anomalous point to dominate the statistic. For this reason, where one or more obvious outliers exists, it is generally better to use ρ than r.

An alternative strategy is to drop the outliers from the data. Careful examination of the anomalous case, and possible reasons for the anomaly, may produce acceptable grounds for doing this. If this course is followed here, we find for data set 2 that $r = .97$ and $\rho = .96$. For data set 3, $r = -.38$ and $\rho = -.32$. Note the huge effect on r of removing the outlier, and the comparatively mild effect on ρ. The various values are summarised in Figure 8.10.

		Data set 1	Data set 2	Data set 3
Full	r	.76	.76	.76
data	ρ	.79	.93	$-.01$
Without	r		.97	$-.38$
outlier	ρ		.96	$-.32$

Figure 8.10 r and ρ data for data sets with identical summary statistics

TESTING FOR SIGNIFICANCE

As with other statistics, r and ρ can be tested for statistical significance. The null hypothesis for r is that *no linear relationship (positive or negative) exists between the*

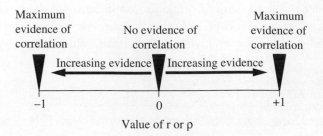

Figure 8.11 Value of r or ρ and strength of evidence

variables (note the specific reference to *linear* relationship, as already discussed). Similarly, the null hypothesis for ρ is that *no general pattern of agreement (positive) or disagreement (negative) between the rankings exists*. In both cases, a value of 0 represents no evidence of a relationship, and the further away from 0 towards either +1 or −1, the stronger the evidence of a relationship, summarised graphically in Figure 8.11.

As usual, a procedure is needed to decide how far from zero r needs to be to be significant. Again, we use a simulation to throw some light on this question. The scatterplot in Figure 8.12 represents a population of 100 cases, with r = ρ = 0; that is, for this population the null hypothesis for both statistics is true. What we do now is to pick ten points at random from this population, shown as black dots in Figure 8.12. For these ten points, r = .06 and ρ = .20. Now we select a different random sample of ten, repeat the process, and so on. . . . The results of twenty such samplings are shown in the form of histograms for the values of r and ρ

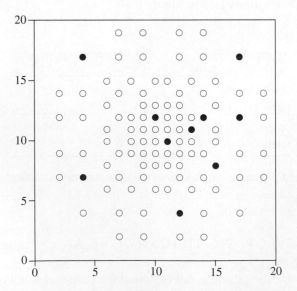

Figure 8.12 Random sample of ten participants from a population with r and ρ = 0

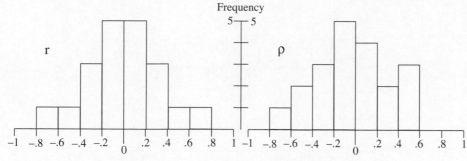

Distributions of values produced by simulation ($N = 10$)

Figure 8.13 Histogram of twenty random samples of ten participants from a population with r and $\rho = 0$

obtained (Figure 8.13). The differences in the histograms reflects the differences in the values of r and ρ. Notice that:

■   the values are roughly symmetrical about zero (in the case of the values for r, the histogram is, in fact, exactly symmetrical 'by chance'); and

■   quite high correlations can be obtained by chance.

Now we repeat the simulation, but with samples of forty participants this time. Figure 8.14 presents the corresponding histograms for twenty samples. Notice that the values cluster much more closely around zero (the same scale was maintained for the histograms to make this obvious). Values beyond ±.2 are relatively unlikely.

As with other statistics, the exact sampling distributions for r and for ρ can be worked out mathematically. In particular, it can be shown that, if the null hypothesis is true for r, and the number of cases, $N = 10$, then the probability of r being as far away from 0 as ±.63 is .05. This statement translates into saying that a value of r (with $N = 10$) greater than .63 or less than −.63 is statistically significant at the .05 level.

The corresponding critical values for ρ are ±.65 (just slightly different). For $N = 40$, the critical values are ±.31 for both r and ρ (see Figure 8.15). The marked difference between $N = 10$ and $N = 40$ confirms the pattern indicated by the simulation – for a small number of cases, there is a much higher chance of a sample 'just by chance' producing a high positive or negative correlation, even though the correlation for the population is zero. The larger the number of cases, the lower this chance becomes, so that a less extreme value of r or ρ is required to reach statistical significance.

In practice, we assume you will be using a statistical package that will tell you if the result is statistically significant or not. It is likely, in fact, that an exact probability will be reported – for example, for $N = 40$ and r = .324, the associated probability is .041 (to 3 decimal places). As this p value is less than .05, the result is statistically significant at the .05 level.

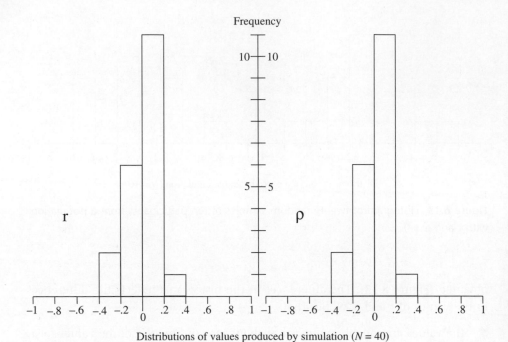

Distributions of values produced by simulation (*N* = 40)

Figure 8.14 Histogram of twenty random samples of forty participants from a population with r and ρ = 0

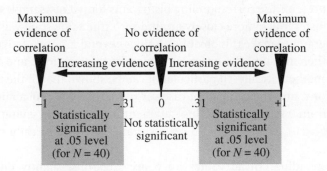

Figure 8.15 Value of r and ρ, and strength of evidence – critical value and statistical significance (*N* = 40)

CORRELATION AND CAUSATION

In many situations where some variable *X causes* another variable, *Y*, it follows that the more of *X*, the more of *Y* (or in some cases, the direction will be reversed – the more of *X*, the less of *Y* – as in the proverbial 'more haste, less speed'). For example, it seems pretty clear that pollution is likely to be a cause of lung disease. This is reflected in data showing that if the level of pollution and the prevalence of lung disease are measured for many different cities, then the values of those two variables will be correlated.

The converse does not necessarily follow. For example, when data began to emerge showing tobacco consumption and lung cancer to be correlated, this did not constitute *logical proof* that smoking causes lung cancer. Apologists for the tobacco industry could argue validly that smokers differ from non-smokers in many ways. For example, it is a logical possibility, however implausible, that smokers generally differ in their personalities in ways that make them more likely to get lung cancer. Or, it may be that smoking is more associated with living in cities, where pollution is higher. Thus, a number of possible alternative explanations could be found for the correlation other than a direct causative link between smoking and lung cancer. On the other hand, it was perfectly reasonable for people concerned about health to argue that the observed correlation is certainly consistent with a causative explanation or, to put it more strongly, suggestive of a causative explanation. In the case of tobacco smoking, the suggestiveness of the correlations was a major motivating factor behind the medical research that identified the underlying causes of lung cancer and proved that tobacco is a factor.

The situation is radically different when the experiment has *direct control*. For example, if animals are tested with a chemical, the experimenter can *randomly assign* animals to different levels of the chemical. If the incidence of a disease rises systematically with the dosage level, this is strong direct evidence that the chemical causes the disease.

Figure 8.16 illustrates an important contrast between situations where a correlation results from X causing Y, and situations where X and Y both have the same underlying (or *latent*) cause (let's call it A). For example, among a sample of people there will clearly be a high correlation between the size of their hands and the size of their feet. Here the variable underlying both of these is general size. In other cases, more complex chains of causation may be hypothesised. For example, it might be speculated that an underlying cause, A, may cause B and C, which in turn cause X and Y respectively, hence accounting for a correlation between X and Y.

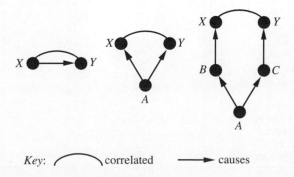

Key: ⌒ correlated   → causes

Figure 8.16 Correlation, causation and latent variables

What can be stated validly is that, if an experimenter hypothesises some link between X and Y in a causative chain, collects data and finds that X and Y are indeed correlated, this may be taken as *some degree* of evidence in support of the hypothesis.

EXAMPLE: BURT'S DATA ON JUVENILE DELINQUENCY

In the 1920s, Sir Cyril Burt studied 'juvenile delinquency' in London. As part of his analysis he compiled a table showing, for each of the twenty-nine boroughs in London, the incidence of juvenile delinquency, and various measures of social conditions, part of which is reproduced in Figure 8.17.

The precise definition of the variables in the table is as follows:

BOROUGH	JUVENILE DELINQUENCY (PER 10 000)	POVERTY (BOOTH'S MEASURE)	POOR RELIEF (PER 1000)	PERCENTAGE OVERCROWDING
Finsbury	42	37	22	34
Holborn	36	49	16	20
Shoreditch	28	42	51	32
Bermondsey	23	44	46	23
St. Pancras	21	30	20	22
Southwark	18	49	32	24
Stepney	17	38	20	29
Battersea	16	38	43	12
Deptford	16	40	40	13
St. Marylebone	15	27	8	18
Westminster	15	35	5	10
Paddington	14	22	15	15
Bethnal Green	14	45	25	28
Islington	14	31	26	19
Hammersmith	13	34	17	14
Lambeth	12	26	21	13
Poplar	12	36	83	21
Kensington	12	25	10	17
Chelsea	12	25	13	14
Greenwich	11	37	16	14
Camberwell	10	29	34	13
Fulham	9	25	14	13
Woolwich	9	25	27	8
Hackney	8	24	18	12
Lewisham	7	18	23	5
City of London	5	32	4	7
Wandsworth	4	27	8	7
Hampstead	2	14	3	7
Stoke Newington	0	19	8	8

Figure 8.17 Burt's data on 'juvenile delinquency', poverty, poor relief and overcrowding

Juvenile delinquency

Number of reported cases per 10 000 of the total number of children on the school rolls during 1922 and 1923.

Poverty

Calculated on the basis of an earlier survey by an experimenter called Charles Booth.

Poor relief

Number per 1000 in receipt of domiciliary relief.

Overcrowding

Percentage of total population living in conditions classified as overcrowded.

(In passing, since all the boroughs of London were included, it could be pointed out that these data are for the whole population (of boroughs), not a sample. However, it could be considered as a sample (though not a random sample, of course) from a larger population of city areas. The analysis of correlation which follows is not affected, in any case.)

To analyse the data in the table, the scatterplots, Product-Moment correlations, and Rank-Order correlations are first produced (see Figure 8.18). The six scatter-grams (representing all possible pairings of the four variables) are arranged in two groups of three. The first column shows the three correlations among Poverty, Poor Relief, and Overcrowding. Each of these may plausibly be considered as a reflection of an underlying variable, namely bad social conditions. The relationship between any two of them is, in a sense, symmetrical (analogous to the relationship between two siblings). It is arbitrary as to which variable is plotted on the horizontal, and which on the vertical, axis.

The second column of three scattergrams represent the correlations of Juvenile Delinquency with each of the three indices of poverty in turn. Here we may at least postulate that Poverty, Poor Relief and Overcrowding are contributory factors in Juvenile Delinquency (it wouldn't make sense to postulate the converse). So the relationships in this case are asymmetrical (like the relationship between a parent and a child, by way of analogy). Conventionally, we plot the possible causal variable on the horizontal axis.

The scatterplots involving Poor Relief show up obvious outliers, and we can trace these to the anomalously high Poor Relief of 83 per cent in Poplar. The correlation coefficients are given with the scatterplots (figures in brackets are for the values of r with the outlier removed). Note, in particular, how the Rank-Order correlation coefficient is much higher for Poor Relief/Juvenile Delinquency; the Product-Moment correlation is much reduced by the outlier, as is indicated by the effect of recalculating it without the outlier.

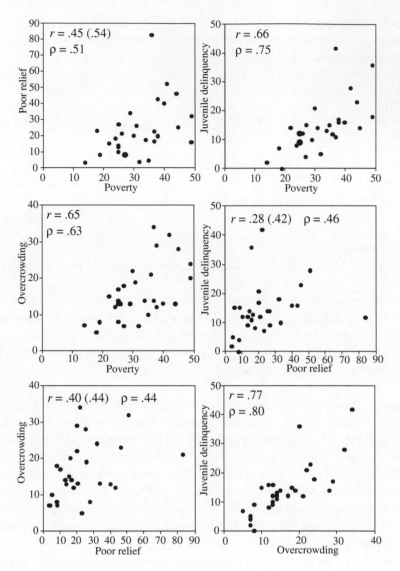

Figure 8.18 Scatterplots, r and ρ for Burt data

Burt's comments on these data are worth quoting:

The highest coefficient of all is that for the correlation between juvenile delinquency and over-crowding, namely .77. Allowing for the gross shortcomings, inevitable in estimates so crude, so vague, and in some cases so largely out of date, these several figures are remarkably consistent one with another. They indicate plainly that it is in the poor, overcrowded, insanitary house-holds . . . that juvenile delinquency is most rife.

But throughout I must insist that, however extensive and however exact, a mere comparison of tabulated figures must never take the place of concrete studies, or of an intensive first-hand scrutiny of the concrete chain of causation, as it operates in particular cases. Here as elsewhere, in gauging the effect of any natural agency, we can put little faith in arm-chair deductions: we must watch that agency at work.

This is an eloquent statement of the principle that, however suggestive correlations may be of causal patterns, they are not by themselves conclusive. He also reminds us that, while general patterns are, of course, important – and the focus of most research in experimental psychology – each individual case is different. Elsewhere in his book, Burt emphasises the multiplicity of factors underlying any such complex social phenomenon, and argues that hereditary and environment explanations are complementary (this, of course, represents one of the deepest questions in psychology).

FITTING A STRAIGHT LINE

The two correlation coefficients we have considered each is a measure, in its own way, of the strength of the relationship between two variables. A further quantification of the relationship is to fit a straight line to the data.

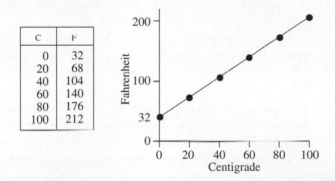

C	F
0	32
20	68
40	104
60	140
80	176
100	212

Figure 8.19 Relationship between Fahrenheit and Centigrade temperatures

By way of introduction to this idea, consider a case where, by definition, an exact straight-line relationship exists, namely temperature measured in Centigrade versus temperature measured in Fahrenheit. Figure 8.19 presents a table and graph showing some such data. The straight line through the points represents the total relationship. Moreover, it can be expressed alternatively in algebraic terms in the equation:

$$F = 32 + 1.8\,C$$

(where F is the temperature in Fahrenheit and C is the temperature in Centigrade). Given any temperature in Centigrade, this formula can be used to work out the corresponding temperature in Fahrenheit.

The general equation for a straight line is:

$$y = a + bx$$

In this equation, a is the value of y when $x = 0$ (see Figure 8.20): it is called the **intercept**, because in graphical terms, it is where the line cuts the y-axis; b is the

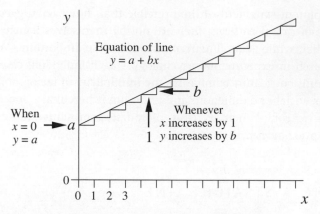

Figure 8.20 Slope, intercept and general equation of straight line

amount y increases by for each unit increase in x – it is called the **slope** (because it determines the slope of the line once the scales for the two axes have been fixed).

By way of an analogy, suppose you hire a car and the charge is £8 initial payment + £35 per day. Then the cost, c, in pounds for n days is given by the formula:

$$c = 8 + 35n$$

Here the initial payment of £8 is like the intercept. The daily payment of £35 is like the slope – for every extra day, the cost increases by another £35.

With psychological data, of course, you just won't get the exact relationship between variables as exists by definition in the Centigrade/Fahrenheit and car-hire examples. Nevertheless, a straight line can be fitted which reflects any trend in the data. To illustrate how this works, consider a very small data set for two variables, labelled X and Y in Figure 8.21.

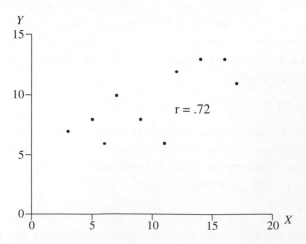

Figure 8.21 Scatterplot of correlated data

The scatterplot shows a fairly strong relationship. It would be possible to fit a straight line 'by eye'; that is, to draw a straight line that best fits the points subjectively. However, it is easy to be more precise. One standard method works by the following line of reasoning. Suppose a particular line is drawn – how could you measure how well it fits the points? A commonly used measure is to take the vertical distance each point lies away from the line, square that, and add them all together. This total, then, is an overall measure of how well the line fits. The **best fit**, by this method of measuring goodness of fit, is clearly the line that makes this value as small as possible. This is called the **regression line**, based on the criterion of so-called **least squares**, i.e., minimizing the sum of the squared vertical distances of the points from the line. Figure 8.22 shows a way of describing schematically the sum of squared vertical distances of the points from a particularly line – the squared distances are represented, literally, as squares.

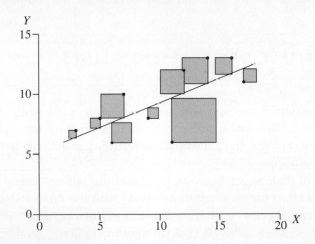

Figure 8.22 Fitting a line using least squares

It is a matter of mathematics to work out the formula for the regression line. Its slope is given by:

$$b = \frac{\sum (X - \overline{X})(Y - \overline{Y})}{\sum (X - \overline{X})^2}$$

and its intercept by:

$$a = \overline{Y} - b\overline{X}$$

For the example, this gives the equation

$$Y' = 5.23 + .42X$$

Note our notation here. Y is used to indicate the actual data values for that variable. Y' we are using to give the equation of the straight line that fits the points on the scattergram, as shown in Figure 8.23.

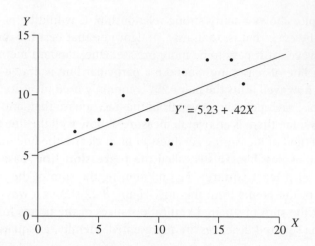

Figure 8.23 Equation of line – slope and intercept calculated from formulae

AN EXAMPLE OF REGRESSION LINES: ANALYSIS OF BURT DATA

As a further example, we apply regression analysis to some of the Burt data already considered. The least-squares regression lines for the relationships between Poverty, Poor Relief and Overcrowding, respectively, and Juvenile Delinquency, are as shown in Figure 8.24.

In the case of Poor Relief, it seems clear that the outlier (Poplar) is having a very distorting effect on the regression line. As with the Product-Moment correlation coefficient, the least-squares method of calculating a line is highly non-resistant; that is, liable to be affected strongly by outliers. One response would be to recalculate the regression line with the outlier omitted, and this leads to a line that appears to summarise more adequately the general trend (Figure 8.25).

Another possible response is to use a rank-based procedure to calculate a line of best fit that is resistant. Figure 8.26 shows how to work out the Tukey line (named after its inventor, John Tukey) for these data:

1 Divide the data vertically into three roughly numerically equal sub-groups – in this case, sub-groups of 10, 9, 10 would be reasonable.

2 For the top sub-group, calculate the median of the values for each variable. For Poor Relief this comes to 37, and for Juvenile Delinquency, 15. Plot these two values as the point (37, 15).

3 Repeat this process for the bottom third of the data, yielding the point (8, 10.5).

4 The line joining these two points determines the slope of the Tukey line. The slope of the line joining two points (x_1, y_1) and (x_2, y_2) in general is $(y_2 - y_1)/(x_2 - x_1)$, so in this case it comes to $b = 4.5/29 = .155$

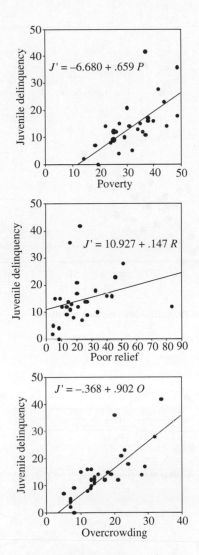

Figure 8.24 Scatterplots and least squares regressions for Burt data

5   In geometrical terms, what is done now is to keep the slope constant, and adjust the line up or down till half of the points lie above it and half below (with 29 points, in fact, it will pass through 1 point and have 14 above and 14 below). In numerical terms, this is achieved by working out $Y - bX$ for each point, and taking the median of these values, which in this case is 9.966. This median defines the intercept, a, so the Tukey line is as shown.

Unfortunately, many pieces of software do not offer this option and, as you can see, it is takes some calculation to work it out. We include it in line with our general policy of stressing resistant statistics.

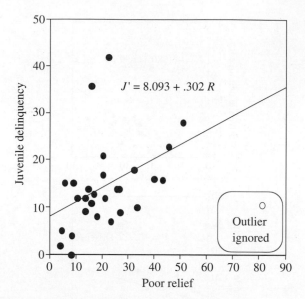

Figure 8.25 Regression recalculated with outlier removed

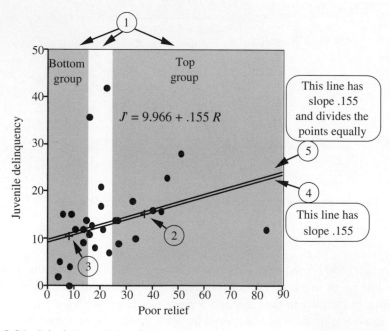

Figure 8.26 Calculating a Tukey line

TESTING FOR SIGNIFICANCE OF REGRESSION

The null hypothesis in this context is that there is *no linear relationship between the variables*. Testing for statistical significance in this case is, in fact, exactly equivalent to testing for the statistical significance of the Product-Moment correlation coefficient.

For example, in the Burt example above, the Product-Moment correlation (r) for Juvenile Delinquency and Poor Relief is .42 with the outlier removed, which for $n = 28$ is highly statistically significant (the critical value is .31). By contrast, the Product-Moment correlation with the outlier included is only .28, which is not statistically significant.

CHAPTER REVIEW

In this chapter, two correlation coefficients have been defined as measures of specific aspects of the relationship between two variables. The Product-Moment Correlation Coefficient is a measure of how closely the data conform to a straight-line relationship, whereas the Rank-Order Correlation Coefficient is a measure of the level of agreement between the two sets of scores when they are ranked. Neither coefficient is equipped to pick up all forms of systematic relationship between two variables – a U-shaped relationship being a case in point. The Rank-Order correlation is resistant by comparison with the Product-Moment coefficient, and is often to be preferred when there is one or more outliers.

These correlation coefficients were illustrated by a number of examples, including data by Burt linking amount of Juvenile Delinquency to indices of unfavourable social conditions. A distinction was made between symmetrical situations in which the variables may be considered as simply related, and asymmetrical situations, in which one variable may be considered as, at least possibly, causing the other. The importance of analysing the relationship between correlation and causation logically was stressed.

A second quantitative approach is to calculate a line that summarises any linear trend in the data. The most common such line is based on minimising the sum of squares of the vertical distances between the points and the line. This is also non-resistant, and can be affected strongly by outliers, so a rank-based alternative was also introduced.

9 Experimentation in psychology

IN THIS CHAPTER
. . .

... through dialogues and the elaboration of earlier examples, ideas about the experimental method introduced in Chapter 1 are extended. Three main experimental designs are discussed – independent groups, repeated measures and matched pairs. Key concepts relating to statistical inference are explored, and linkages between experimental design and choice of statistical test are made explicit.

PUTTING A LITTLE MORE MEAT ON THE BONES

In the preceding chapters, we have presented many important statistical and methodological concepts. Here, we pull these ideas together. By integrating various concepts, the inextricable links between research design and statistical methods are made explicit.

Inevitably, this chapter will involve cross-referencing to earlier material. In order to reduce the amount of scuttling back and forth, we reiterate the essential details of the various examples as appropriate.

RECAP: THE EMPIRICAL PROCESS

Figure 9.1 summarises the elements of the empirical approach first introduced in Chapter 1 (see page 10). Recall that the researcher defines a topic, identifies specific hypotheses and then designs a study to generate data intended to cast light on these hypotheses. Following statistical analysis of the data, findings are interpreted, disseminated and integrated into existing knowledge.

In this chapter, we focus on the approach known as the experimental method, first discussed in Chapter 1 (see page 11). As we explained there, the essence of experimental studies is the control, or manipulation, of so-called **independent**

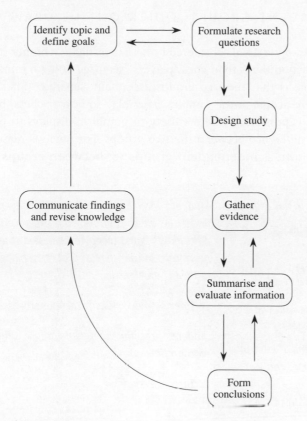

Figure 9.1 The empirical process

variables – a characteristic that allows causal relationships between variables to be investigated.

EXPERIMENTAL DESIGNS

For the sake of clarity, and consistent with our approach, we recap and draw together the ideas about experimental design introduced in earlier chapters. In keeping with our philosophy, we consider at this point only the basic forms of experimental design.

DESIGNS FOR COMPARING TWO SETS OF SCORES

In Chapter 7 you were introduced to statistical tests for comparing scores, based on either two separate groups of participants, or on testing the same individuals on two occasions. Let's look in a little more detail at the design of the experiments from which such data originate.

INDEPENDENT GROUPS: QUICK ON THE DRAW

Recall that in Chapter 4 we considered how to investigate whether squash players have faster reaction times than chess players (see page 50). An important feature of this example is that the two groups are totally separate (for simplicity, we assume that the people in the samples *either* play squash *or* chess, but not both). As we saw, it is possible to use a variety of graphical displays to provide visual evidence of a difference between the two groups. For obvious reasons, this type of design is known as **independent groups** (or **between groups**).

Lecturer: What are the main variables in this example?

Student: Let's see, one variable is whether someone is a squash player or a chess player.

Lecturer: That's right, but do you know what type of variable it is?

Student: Er... an independent variable with two levels – squash and chess?

Lecturer: It certainly has two levels and it's an independent variable of sorts – but what more can you say about it?

Student: Ah, yes, it's a subject variable, because it's not under the direct control of the experimenter. So, when participants come along to be tested, they are already designated as squash players or chess players – that's one of their characteristics.

Lecturer: Good. Now, is there another variable?

Student: Yes, the dependent variable is the participants' reaction time.

Lecturer: Well done!

MORE ON INDEPENDENT GROUPS: CHANGING COMPUTER ATTITUDES

Chapter 7 presents another independent groups design, in which one group of ten females is shown a video intended to foster positive attitudes towards computers, while a separate group of ten females is not shown the video.

BEFORE READING ON . . .

Look back at this example. Name the independent and dependent variables.

. . . now read on

In this example, the independent variable, let's call it *Condition*, is manipulated at two levels – *video/no-video*, and participants are assigned randomly to one of the two treatments. The *video* group may be referred to as an **experimental group**, while the *no-video* group is one example of a **control group**.

The precise nature of the control condition is an important matter in itself. For example, instead of a *no-video* control, we could opt for a control treatment in which participants are shown a neutral video (for example, about natural history) of the same duration. You may consider this to be a more appropriate control, since it is more similar to the experimental task than the *no-video* control.

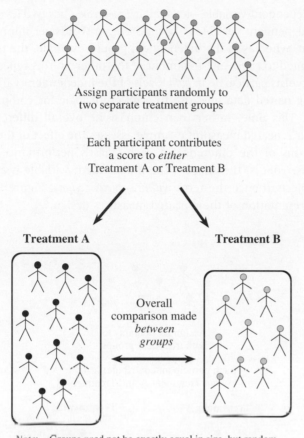

Assign participants randomly to
two separate treatment groups

Each participant contributes
a score to *either*
Treatment A or Treatment B

Treatment A   **Treatment B**

Overall
comparison made
*between
groups*

Note: Groups need not be exactly equal in size, but random
assignment should ensure roughly similar group sizes

Figure 9.2 Independent (or between) groups design

The dependent variable is the measure of *Computer Attitudes*. As you saw in Chapter 7, the effect of watching the video on the dependent variable is assessed by comparing the *overall* performance of the two groups. Put another way, the comparison is made *between* groups (hence, the term *between groups design*). A schematic representation of the between groups design is given in Figure 9.2.

PAIRED DATA: LET YOUR FINGERS DO THE TALKING

Chapter 7 presents an example of a **repeated measures** (or **within-subjects**) design, in which the typing speed of a single group of sixteen typists is measured on two occasions – before and after a tea-break (see page 114).

BEFORE READING ON . . .

What are the independent and dependent variables in this example?

. . . now read on

Here the independent variable – let's call it *Tea-break* – has two levels – *before* and *after*, and the dependent variable is *Typing Speed*, in words per minute. It is worth reiterating that, whereas in the independent groups example, the twenty participants are assigned to *either* one treatment *or* the other, in this repeated measures example, the typists participate in *both* levels of the independent variable.

The resulting paired data give rise to a different logic for comparing the two sets of scores. This time, rather than emphasising overall differences between treatments, our repeated measures example assesses the effect of the independent variable in terms of the difference in each typist's performance between the two treatments. That is, the effect of the independent variable is assessed *within* individual subjects (hence the term *within-subjects design*). Figure 9.3 presents a schematic representation of the repeated measures design.

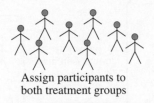

Assign participants to
both treatment groups

Each participant contributes a score
to *both* Treatment A and Treatment B

Treatment A   **Treatment B**

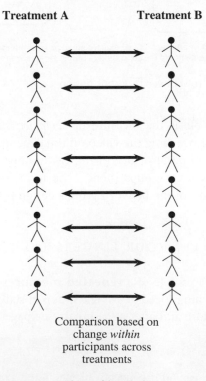

Comparison based on
change *within*
participants across
treatments

Figure 9.3 Repeated measures (or within-subjects) design

MATCHED PAIRS: BOYS' AND GIRLS' MATHEMATICAL ABILITIES

In Chapter 7, we presented another case of paired data, although that time the design also involved separate groups of participants. You might rightly regard it as a hybrid between independent groups and repeated measures. Recall that, in

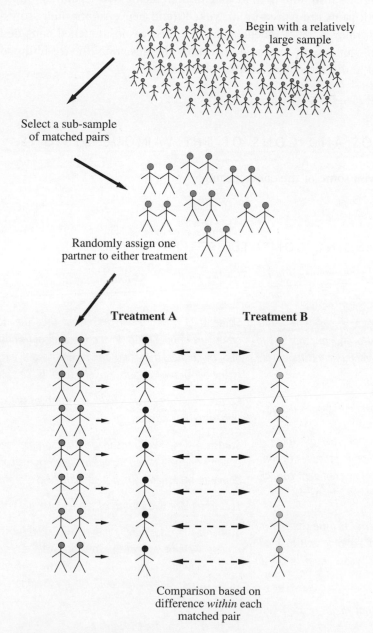

Begin with a relatively large sample

Select a sub-sample of matched pairs

Randomly assign one partner to either treatment

Treatment A   Treatment B

Comparison based on difference *within* each matched pair

Figure 9.4 Matched pairs design

this example of a **matched pairs design**, initial samples of boys and girls are *pre-tested* for intelligence and then a sub-sample of boy–girl pairs with matched IQs are chosen. Here the independent variable is gender at two levels; the dependent variable is mathematical ability; and the **matching variable** is IQ. Obviously, since gender is a subject variable, participants cannot be assigned randomly to the levels of the independent variable! A schematic representation of the matched pairs design is shown in Figure 9.4.

It is important to note that, in spite of there being two separate groups, the fact that participants are paired-up or 'yoked' (and hence so are their scores) means that the groups are not independent. For this reason, matched pairs designs are classified along with repeated measures designs, and the resulting data are analysed in the same way as other paired data.

PROS AND CONS OF THE VARIOUS DESIGNS

Let's revisit some of the above examples.

CHANGING COMPUTER ATTITUDES (AGAIN)

Lecturer: Think about our example, in which one group of females is shown a video and another group isn't, and then both groups' computer attitudes are measured.

Student: I remember, the independent groups design.

Lecturer: That's right. Suppose that, overall, those in the video condition have more positive attitudes to computers than the no-video group. How confident can you be that the difference is caused by the video?

Student: Depending on the size of the difference, pretty confident. The independent variable was manipulated by the experimenter, so I can infer a causal relationship.

Lecturer: Are there any issues that might cause you to hesitate?

Student: I suppose if I discovered that the no-video group just happened to have a few radical technophobes and, by chance, the video group contained five members of the Bill Gates fan club, I might think twice.

Lecturer: What do you think the chances are of something like that happening?

Student: OK. Well, assuming the samples were big enough and the experimenter assigned participants randomly to treatments, then it shouldn't be a problem.

Lecturer: Are two groups of ten females big enough?

Student: I'm not sure – maybe. It's quite possible the groups weren't equivalent to start with, even if they were randomly selected, and one or two 'extreme' individuals in either group could tip the balance in either direction.

Lecturer: Food for thought, eh?

LET YOUR FINGERS DO THE TALKING (AGAIN)

Let's look again at the *Tea-break* example. Clearly, there is no problem with non-equivalent groups. Not only are the groups equivalent – they are identical, with each typist acting as her or his own control. So, supposing typing speed is faster after a tea-break, can we be more confident this time that the difference results from the independent variable?

BEFORE READING ON . . .

Think about this question and jot down your thoughts.

. . . now read on

Student: I think I might know the answer, because I had some doubts when we analysed this example in Chapter 7. As I see it, the problem stems from the fact that, since each typist undergoes both treatments, by definition, they must do so sequentially.

Lecturer: Why might that cause a problem?

Student: Well, say the typists just got better due to practice, or getting warmed up, or becoming more relaxed about being tested – any of these might cause an improvement in performance after the tea-break. On the other hand, say they became increasingly tired, or bored, or anxious – any of these might worsen performance, thus underestimating the benefits of a tea-break. I dare say there are a hundred other possibilities.

Lecturer: Good answer. Whether you are aware of it or not, you have identified the main disadvantage of repeated measures designs. Depending on what book you read, or whom you talk to, you will find them referred to as **order**, **transfer** or **range effects**.

Student: Is there any way of overcoming these problems?

Lecturer: Fortunately, yes.

COPING WITH TRANSFER

There are two broad approaches to dealing with order effects in repeated measures designs. One is to find some way to minimise **transfer** from the first condition to the second. The other, more common, approach is to **alternate** or **counterbalance** the order of conditions across participants.

In fact, everyday life is full of examples of alternating conditions. Sport is a particularly rich vein, given the obvious need to ensure that one competitor does not have an advantage over another. In tennis, players swap sides every two games throughout a match. In chess, players take turns between white and black. In sports such as soccer, ice hockey, field hockey, basketball and rugby, teams change ends at half-time, or at the end of each quarter. Similarly, in knock-out competitions, the result of a tie may be taken over two legs – home and away.

The instinct to balance any possible advantage of one competitor over another is ever-present, even when we cannot necessarily identify the precise nature of any advantage. Beyond the sporting arena, we find other everyday examples. You may be familiar with the advice to turn houseplants regularly through 180 degrees to ensure even growth. We are also told that swapping the front and rear tyres on your car every 6000 miles will promote even wear across the life of the tyres.

BEFORE READING ON . . .

Try to identify some more real-life examples of alternating treatments of conditions. Jot these down for later discussion with friends or your tutor.

. . . now read on

LET YOUR FINGERS DO THE TALKING (AGAIN)

Back to our *Tea-break* experiment. In this case, one option for dealing with order effects is to try to minimise the impact of transfer from *before* to *after*.

BEFORE READING ON . . .

Spend some time thinking about how you could cope with order effects in this example. Jot down your thoughts for later comparison.

. . . now read on

Let's see how you got on. One method of dealing with the problem would be to increase the time interval between conditions, so that order effects are minimised. For example, the *before* condition could be done on one day (with no *after* testing) and the *after* condition done the next (with no *before* testing). That way, many (but not all) of the order effects would be reduced. Incidentally, this approach would also allow half of the participants to do *after* on the first day, followed by *before* on the next, and vice versa.

BEFORE READING ON . . .

Which of the following might be minimised by this method:

- practice;

- anxiety;

- boredom;'

- memory of the content of the test;

- fatigue; or

- getting warmed up?

Any others you can think of?

. . . now read on

ALTERNATING TREATMENTS

Fortunately, unlike the *Tea-break* example, most repeated measures designs do not require treatments to be carried out in a rigid sequence. For example, suppose we are interested in comparing memory for written and spoken words. We could carry out a repeated measures experiment by exposing participants to two sets of words – one written, the other spoken, and testing memory for each. Half of the group would be randomly selected to take *written* followed by *spoken*, while the remainder would do the opposite. Figure 9.5 shows this approach more generally – a simple example of the **Latin Square Design**.

Student: Cool! So, when the data are aggregated for the whole group, any transfer from the first to the second condition will be balanced by an equivalent transfer in the opposite direction.

Lecturer: Correct, although the assumption that transfer is symmetrical, that is, that one direction cancels out the other, is precisely that – an assumption.

Student: Also, even if transfer does cancel out across the whole group, for any individual participant, the transfer effects remain.

Lecturer: Indeed, so if you want to look at a single participant, or a very small group, alternating treatments might not be suitable.

Student: Then what?

Lecturer: Let's see.

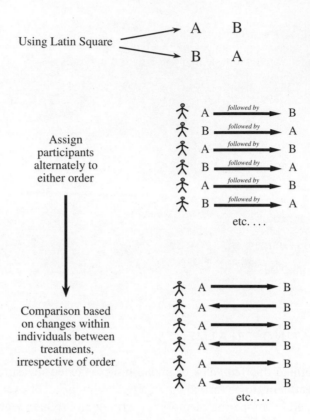

Figure 9.5 Latin Square Design

COUNTERBALANCING: A–B–B–A

Another method of alternating treatments, known as counterbalancing, is to ask participants to perform the first treatment . . . followed by the second . . . followed by the second again . . . followed by the first (see Figure 9.6). So, in the case of our memory example, participants would take (say) *written* first, *spoken* second, *spoken* third and *written* fourth.

Averages are then obtained for each participant's two *written* scores and two *spoken* scores. The logic here is that any order effects are balanced out because participants do one treatment first and last, and the other treatment second and third. An assumption here is that such transfer applies *evenly* across the four conditions, for example, in the case of a gradual build up of fatigue or reduction of anxiety. Again, this assumption may not always hold.

The advantage of this method is that the order effects are controlled for each participant, so it is not necessary to average over an entire group to see the benefit. This is particularly useful if the number of participants is limited. However, the

All participants undergo
both treatments *twice*, in
the following sequence:

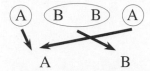

A *followed by* B *followed by* B *followed by* A

Each participant's two
A & B scores are averaged

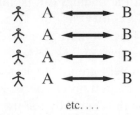

A   B

In the ususal way for repeated
measures, comparison is based on
differences in A & B scores
within each participant

🚶 A ←——→ B
🚶 A ←——→ B
🚶 A ←——→ B
🚶 A ←——→ B

etc. . . .

Figure 9.6 Counterbalancing

disadvantage is that each participant has to perform a total of four conditions, which may be problematic if the tasks are lengthy.

BOYS' AND GIRLS' MATHEMATICAL ABILITIES

Recall the matched pairs example from Chapter 7, in which girl–boy pairs, matched for intelligence, are compared on mathematical ability (see page 119).

Student: This design looks as if it offers the best of both worlds. I can't imagine why psychologists don't use it all the time.

Lecturer: Why do you like it so much?

Student: Well, although you have two separate groups, because participants have been matched and paired up, you also have related scores.

Lecturer: So?

Student: The independent groups ensure that there can be no transfer between conditions – participants are only tested once. Since participants are pre-tested and care-fully matched, although the paired scores are not from the same individual, they might as well be.

Lecturer: Do you think it's as cut and dried as that?

continued

Student:　Well . . . yes. Don't you?

Lecturer:　Often it is pretty cut and dried, but it is important to be aware that the experimenter has to assume that the chosen pre-test is a valid means of matching participants; that is, it must take account of all variables likely to affect performance in the experiment. It should also be borne in mind that the pre-testing of participants is logistically more demanding than independent groups or repeated measures, and may even be impractical.

Student:　Ah, so that's why psychologists don't use it all the time!

SUMMING UP: DESIGN, VALIDITY AND INSIDIOUS VARIABLES

It should be clear to you by now that, in designing experiments, considerable care must be taken to ensure that the findings can be interpreted unambiguously, a property known as **internal validity**. In our discussion of the anatomy of the three main experimental designs, we have identified various threats to internal validity. In the case of independent groups designs, we saw that results may be unclear because of non-equivalent groups. Repeated measures designs, on the other hand, are prone to order and transfer effects, while the internal validity of matched pairs designs may be threatened by the use of an inappropriate matching variable.

The empirical arena is full of **extraneous variables** that affect a participant's behaviour. The majority of these exert a relatively minor, and random, influence, so are simply ignored as so-called **nuisance variables**. Some extraneous variables, however, are more insidious, biasing data systematically and otherwise threatening internal validity. Researchers have developed an impressive armoury of methodological devices to deal with these **confounding variables**, many of which are found in this book. Rather than review these ideas in isolation, we discuss them as an integral part of the statistical techniques they support.

STATISTICAL INFERENCE

In preceding chapters, you will have encountered the idea that, in all but the rarest cases, psychological research involves the use of one or more samples of participants drawn from one or more target populations. The role of statistical tests is to allow us to generalise findings from these samples to their respective populations. Generally, since textbooks have tended to use somewhat arcane, though in most cases technically correct, language to explain this idea, students could be forgiven for struggling to grasp the nub of the issue.

FROM SAMPLE TO POPULATION: THE STORY SO FAR

Chapter 6 used the example of Big-Endians (B) and Little-Endians (L) from *Gulliver's Travels* to illustrate a popular approach to statistical inference involving the *null hypothesis* (see page 88). In this example, the null hypothesis is that Bs and Ls are represented equally in the population. The essence of the approach is to take a sample of the population and count the numbers of Bs and Ls. The likelihood of this result having occurred, assuming equal numbers of Bs and Ls, is then evaluated.

This is a somewhat indirect approach to the precise question of how many Bs and Ls there are in the population. As we pointed out in Chapter 6, our result does *not* tell us how likely it is that there are equal numbers of Bs and Ls. Rather, for the sake of argument, we *assume* equal numbers in the population (that is, that the null hypothesis is true). After counting the number of Bs and Ls in the sample, we then ask, 'What is the likelihood of obtaining such a result, assuming that the null hypothesis is true'.

By convention, if the imbalance between Bs and Ls in the sample is such that the likelihood of it having occurred under the null hypothesis is 5 per cent (.05) or less, we declare the result to be statistically significant, and we decide to *reject* the null hypothesis. On the other hand, if the result is less extreme, such that the likelihood of it occurring under the null hypothesis is greater than this cut-off of .05, we *fail to reject* the null hypothesis. This cut-off point of .05 is known as the **level of significance**, a term introduced in Chapter 6 (see page 91). More of this later.

ERRORS IN STATISTICAL INFERENCE

Self-evidently, in any situation where decisions are taken on the basis of probability, there is a risk – albeit possibly a very small one – of that decision being wrong. Take the example of a jury in a court of law entrusted with the task of reaching a verdict in the absence of total certainty. In such situations, there are two possible decisions – innocent or guilty – and two possible states of reality – innocence or guilt. Of course, in most legal systems, jurisprudence dictates that a defendant is innocent until found to be guilty beyond all reasonable doubt. Figure 9.7 illustrates the relationship between decision and reality, as well as four possible scenarios.

While the outcomes shown in Figure 9.7 may seem obvious, for reasons that will become clear it is worth taking a little time to consider them. Depending on the reality of the situation, namely the guilt or innocence of the defendant, the jury risks making one of two possible errors – either wrongly to convict an innocent person, or wrongly to acquit a guilty person. Bear in mind that the jury are not privy to the reality of the situation. Presuming the defendant to be innocent, they must evaluate the facts of the case and decide whether the evidence casts

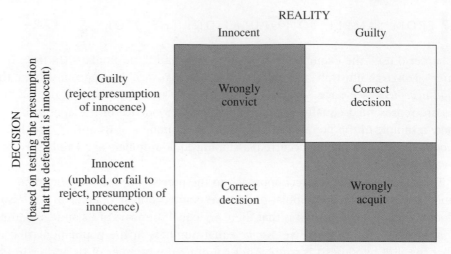

Figure 9.7 Reaching a verdict – four possible outcomes

reasonable doubt on this presumption of innocence. The question, 'How reasonable should *reasonable* be?' also arises. Which outcome is worse – letting a guilty person walk free, or sending an innocent person to jail? Indeed, in some legal systems, the consequence of a wrong conviction may be even more profound.

> **BEFORE READING ON . . .**
>
> Spend some time thinking about these points. Do you notice any parallels with statistical inference in psychology experiments? Jot down your thoughts for later reflection.
>
> *. . . now read on*

This example is a useful analogy for statistical inference in experiments. The presumption that *the defendant is innocent* may be thought of as the null hypothesis. The examination of the facts by the jury is akin to analysis of the data. The jury's consideration of the likelihood of the events occurring, assuming the defendant is innocent, is similar to deciding whether the results of an experiment are significant or not. Only *strong* doubt that the defendant's innocence was consistent with the facts of the case would lead the jury to reject the presumption of innocence – effectively to reject the null hypothesis. If, on the other hand, the jury considered it possible that the events could have occurred, given a presumption of innocence, there would not be grounds to reject the null hypothesis.

Figure 9.8 summarises outcomes in relation to experimental reality and corresponding decisions about the null hypothesis (H_o). As in the jury example, we see that there are two possible types of error in making statistical inferences. First, the researcher could wrongly *reject* the null hypothesis *when it was true* (cf,

REALITY

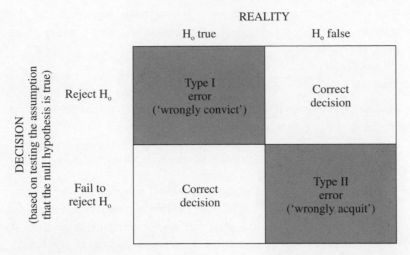

Figure 9.8 Type I and II errors

'wrongly convict an innocent person'), or they could wrongly *fail to reject* the null hypothesis *when it was false* (cf, 'wrongly acquit a guilty person'). Note from Figure 9.8 that these decision errors are called **Type I** and **Type II** errors, respectively.

STATISTICAL SIGNIFICANCE, REASONABLE DOUBT AND TYPE I ERRORS

It should be clear by now that the process of statistical inference involves a gamble. In any experiment, the essence of this approach to statistical analysis of the data is to calculate *the likelihood of obtaining our result, assuming the null hypothesis to be true*. Since the result of this calculation is in the form of a probability, we must then decide whether or not the evidence is strong enough to allow us to reject the null hypothesis.

While in the jury example, their level of confidence was expressed in terms of strong doubt, statistical inference is based on setting firm levels of risk in taking decisions. Earlier in this chapter, we referred to the so-called *.05 level of significance* used widely in psychological research. This cut-off value of .05 (or 5 per cent) is the probability value corresponding to the *likelihood of obtaining a result equal to, or more extreme than our result*.

Student: So, basically, if the probability of obtaining a result as extreme as ours – assuming the null hypothesis to be true – is .05 or less, we consider it doubtful that the null hypothesis could have produced this result?

Lecturer: Correct. If you like, we have set a 5 per cent likelihood as a cut-off for strong doubt, which we call the level of significance.

Student: But sometimes we'll be wrong in rejecting the null hypothesis.

Lecturer: Indeed – after all, it's a game of chance like any other, and that's the risk we take.

Student: So you're saying that 'significant at the 5 per cent level' means that even for a null hypothesis that is true, there is a small chance that the result will be interpreted as statistically significant.

Lecturer: Right.

Student: Ah, I've seen a link that hadn't occurred to me before – the level of significance is the risk of making this mistake.

Lecturer: Exactly. In fact, many statistics texts define level of significance as the probability of wrongly rejecting a true null hypothesis, or words to that effect.

Student: Hang on, I think I see another link. Isn't this type of mistake called a Type I error?

Lecturer: Correct.

Student: So, doing some joined-up thinking, isn't level of significance actually the probability of making a Type I error?

Lecturer: Excellent! You will often see level of significance abbreviated to the Greek letter α – pronounced 'alfa' – in textbooks and computer-based statistical packages.

Student: I'm sure I've also seen it referred to as **p** in some text books.

Lecturer: Actually, α and p are not exactly the same, although they are very closely related. Both represent the level of significance; that is, the probability of wrongly rejecting a true null hypothesis.

Student: So what's the difference?

Lecturer: Well, α is a **predefined** cut-off point, such as .05. So, when you carry out a statistical test, you compare your result with a so-called critical value of the statistic representing your predefined level of significance. Your decision to reject the null hypothesis or not would depend on whether your result is greater or less (depending on the test) than the corresponding critical value.

Student: What is p then?

Lecturer: Unlike α, p is not a predefined cut-off. As we saw in Chapter 7, it is the **precise** significance associated with your result. Since computers came along, it has been possible to calculate exact p values, rather than simply asking whether a result is above or below a cut-off point, such as .05. So, when a statistical test is calculated on a computer, you obtain a p value – such as .004, or .3318, or even .0000 to 4 decimal places – and you simply look to see whether this value is equal to or less than .05, say.

Student: Ah, so you don't need to compare the actual value of the statistic with its corresponding critical value – you just need to look at the p value. That's definitely a handier way to do it, thanks to the good old computer.

Lecturer: But remember, ultimately both approaches tell you the same thing, that is, whether or not you should reject the null hypothesis.

BEFORE READING ON . . .

You may find it useful to look again at Chapter 7 (pages 97, 108–9). Make sure you understand the points raised in the above dialogue and how they relate to those in Chapter 7.

. . . now read on

Student: Mind you, a cut-off of .05 might be an acceptable level of risk in some psychology experiments, but I'm not sure I would always want to risk making wrong decisions 5 per cent of the time. Also, if I were researching a cure for cancer, or trying to send a rocket to the moon, I would want to be much more confident than that.

Lecturer: Indeed – remember that .05 is a cut-off that we deem to be an acceptable level of risk for general purposes. However, we are free to set any value of α that we wish. In fact, an alternative to $\alpha = .05$ adopted in many psychology experiments is to set an α value of .01.

Student: So in these cases, the probability of a Type I error is reduced to 1 per cent?

Lecturer: Right – and in the case of research of the sort you mentioned, with critical consequences, we can reduce the probability of a Type I error as much as we like by setting very small α values, like .005, .001, .0001, and so on.

Student: Cool! But why don't we make the α value as small as we possibly can, so that we virtually never make a Type I error?

Lecturer: There is an important trade-off in doing this, as we shall see.

BEFORE READING ON . . .

Read this dialogue again in conjunction with Figure 9.8. Make sure you can see the various linkages. Can you think what 'trade-off' the lecturer is talking about? Jot down your thoughts.

. . . now read on

STATISTICAL POWER, REASONABLE CONFIDENCE AND TYPE II ERRORS

While reducing the risk of a Type I error may be a laudable objective, this is only one side of a two-sided coin. Consider what happens as a researcher sets lower and lower significance levels. (In a sense, reducing the probability of wrongly rejecting the null hypothesis is achieved at the cost of making it less likely that you will reject the null hypothesis *at all*, whether it is true or false.) While the risk of a Type I error may have been reduced, the corresponding reluctance to reject the null hypothesis increases the risk of retaining a null hypothesis that is, in reality, untrue – that is, the probability of a Type II error.

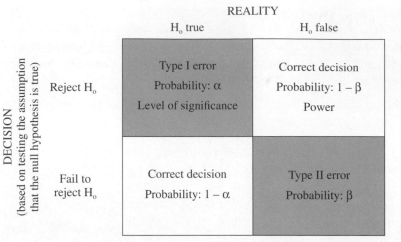

Figure 9.9 Decision errors, significance and power

In research, it is just as desirable to avoid Type II errors as it is to minimise Type I errors. The notion of statistical **power** is closely linked to that of Type II error. Power refers to the *probability that a researcher will reject the null hypothesis when it should be rejected*. Figure 9.9 summarises the various relationships between power, Type II errors and statistical significance. By convention, the probability of a Type II error is denoted by the Greek letter β (pronounced 'bee-ta'), and statistical power by $1 - \beta$.

Student: So, by setting a very small level of significance, the chance of you failing to take seriously a 'real' result is decreased – that is, you reduce power.

Lecturer: Correct. However, it's more a matter of where to set the balance between Type I and Type II errors, as in the question posed earlier in this section – namely, Which is worse – acquitting a guilty person, or convicting an innocent one?

Student: I suppose it depends on the circumstances. If I were a clinical psychologist assessing the effectiveness of a new treatment with potentially harmful side-effects, I'd want to be pretty sure that it worked before cutting loose on my patients – so I would try to minimise the risk of a Type I error. In other circumstances, I may wish to be more speculative and accept a lower standard for statistical significance.

Lecturer: In thinking about this, you might find the following analogy useful. Suppose an astronomer has two telescopes – one quite weak but pretty reliable, the other very powerful but more prone to producing artefacts. Now, this astronomer thinks she may have discovered a new star. If so, she has calculated that it will appear in a particular part of the sky on a given evening. Which telescope would you suggest she uses?

Student: Well, ultimately, it depends on the reality of the situation – but she can't know this in advance.

Lecturer: Take me through the hypothetical scenario that, in reality, there is no new star.

Student: Right, say she assumes there is no star (that is, the null hypothesis is true) – and in reality there isn't one. If she used the powerful telescope and saw some-

thing, she would reject the null hypothesis, but she would have made a Type I error, since it was an aberration. If she used the weaker telescope, she wouldn't see anything, and she'd be right not to reject the null hypothesis.

Lecturer: Now, say there is a new star.

Student: Well, she should still begin with the assumption that there isn't one. Now, if she used the powerful telescope, she would almost certainly see the new star – even if it were quite faint – and she would correctly reject the null hypothesis. On the other hand, if she used this weaker instrument and did not see anything – especially if the star were faint – she would conclude that there was no new star, thus making a Type II error.

Lecturer: I hope you see statistical tests are like telescopes. Some are powerful and others less so. Powerful statistical tests have a greater ability than their more conservative counterparts to find an effect where one exists – even a weak effect. By the same token, they also increase the risk of a false positive; that is, 'detecting' an effect where one does not exist. Less powerful methods reduce the risk of such false positives, but are more likely to miss out, as it were.

FACTORS AFFECTING POWER

Nowadays, it is recommended that you assess the likelihood that your experiment will detect an effect, if one exists, *before* carrying out the research. Power calculations are becoming more prevalent in published research, although they are still far from commonplace. While calculation of power is outside the scope of this book, it is important to have a conceptual grasp of the principles underlying its calculation. Several factors are known to affect statistical power, and these should be addressed when designing a study, whether experimental or observational.

Effect size

It may go without saying that, if an effect exists, then the stronger that effect, the better your chances of detecting it. Thus, in assessing power, you need to get a handle on the magnitude of the effect. This information may be available in previously published research, or it may be calculated, or indeed estimated. There are several approaches to calculating so-called **effect size**, although many of those textbooks that mention the topic tend to portray it as something of a black art. The one we will use is the effect size correlation coefficient.

In the case of correlational studies, i.e. where two or more variables are measured and the strength of the relationship between the variables is calculated using Pearson r, the calculation of effect size is easy – it is simply indicated by the value of r. In experimental studies, however, involving two or more treatment conditions to be compared, another type of correlation coefficient has to be calculated to indicate the magnitude of the effect of the independent variable on the dependent variable. As with all correlaion coefficients, these latter effect sizes also have numerical values between 0 and 1. The important value of these effect size calculations is that, unlike the values of other statistics, they are consistent and therefore provide a common metric across all research designs irrespective of sample size and the types of variable use.

The formula for effect size differs depending on the type of study and we do not propose to deal with this here. Rather than calculate effect size, many researchers find Cohen's benchmark values helpful. This involves the experimenter making a qualitative judgement as to whether the expected size of the effect is 'small', 'medium' or 'large', and on this basis selecting a benchmark value of .1, .3, or .5 respectively. This value can then be used in the calculation of power.

Significance level

As we have already seen, the 'cut-off' α value chosen by the experimenter can have a major effect on statistical power. In short, the more stringent the level of significance, the less power.

Sample size

In preceding chapters, we have considered some of the implications of sample size for statistical tests. Overall, we conclude that larger samples provide better estimates of population values than smaller samples, and are less subject to the effects of outliers and other potentially harmful influences. In the context of statistical power, the larger the sample, the greater the power, which is especially important if effect sizes are moderate.

Choice of statistical test

As a rule of thumb, the so-called *parametric* tests, such as the t-test and Pearson r, are more powerful than their rank-based equivalents. One obvious reason for this is the fact that the former use actual scores in the calculation of the statistic, and so are more sensitive to patterns within the data.

Choice of experimental design

Repeated measures designs tend to be more powerful than equivalent independent groups designs, because of the emphasis they place on changes *within* the same individuals (tested under two conditions), rather than on overall differences *between* separate groups.

TO SUM UP

It is advisable to consider these factors when designing a study. All other things being equal, identify a research question that previous research suggests may offer a reasonable effect size; choose a repeated measures design; recruit as large a sample as possible; don't set your α value any higher than necessary; and, provided assumptions are met, analyse the data using parametric statistics. If only it were that simple!

CHOOSING THE RIGHT STATISTICAL TEST

Saturday, 10.00 am

Salesman: Good day, Madam, can I be of assistance?

Client: I'd like to buy a car, but I'm having trouble making up my mind.

Salesman: I see. Perhaps I can be of some help.

What do you do for a living? (Investment broker)

Do you have a spending figure in mind? (Flexible)

Can I ask if you will be sharing the car with any other drivers? (No)

Do you have any children? (No)

How much driving do you do? (Lots)

What's your favourite colour of car? (Yellow)

What are you looking for in a car? (Sporty, fast, chic)

Perhaps I can interest you in our latest German sports cars brochure. Step this way, Madam.

Saturday, 10.25 am

Salesman: Good day, Madam, can I be of assistance?

Client: I'd like to buy a car, but I'm having trouble making up my mind.

Salesman: I see. Perhaps I can be of some help.

What do you do for a living? (Parent)

Do you have spending figure in mind? (Not exactly, but limited)

Can I ask if you will be sharing the car with any other drivers? (My partner)

Do you have any children? (Five)

How much driving do you do? (Shops and schools mostly)

What's your favourite colour of car (Anything that's not rusted)

What are you looking for in a car? (Cheap, space for 2 adults, 5 kids, 2 dogs and can tow a caravan)

Ah, yes. I think there may be something out the back. Step this way, Madam. I don't know if you've heard, but converted second-hand buses are all the rage these days.

'What has this got to do with choosing statistical tests?' we hear you ask. Well, when choosing a new car, we find there are lots of different, models, types, colours, prices – many more than there are statistical tests in fact. Cars all do roughly the same thing – they get you from A to B. Some differences between models are major, some are merely subtle nuances, others are technical. In spite of the choice being difficult at times, few people would argue that there should be fewer models of car from which to choose.

Contrast this with statistical tests. Students often claim to find the number and variety of statistical tests confusing: 'How do I decide which one to choose on any given occasion?' they exclaim. 'Why can't there just be one or two tests?' Sound familiar?

We agree that there do appear to be a lot of statistical tests and it's not always easy to choose between them. Try to think of it as a bit like choosing a car. Just as different cars suit different circumstances, in deciding upon a suitable statistical test, you have to take into account a number of factors.

WHAT DO WE KNOW SO FAR?

In the first eight chapters of this book, we introduced and discussed all the ideas and concepts needed to inform your choice of statistical technique for simple experimental designs, whether it be for summarising, displaying or analysing data. In Chapter 2 we presented a series of examples of methods used by psychologists to measure behaviour, and went on to consider the properties of the data generated by these methods. We discussed the characteristics of performance measures (dependent variables) in terms of their *levels of measurement* (nominal, ordinal, interval or ratio). We also considered briefly variables under experimental control (independent variables).

In Chapter 3, we discussed different methods for summarising and displaying single data sets, depending on the properties of the variable and the summary information required. We then elaborated these ideas in Chapters 4 and 5 to include comparisons, and relationships between two variables. Chapters 7 and 8 further extended this approach to include statistical methods for comparing and relating data.

Recall that, in Chapter 3, we discussed how the properties of our variable influence our choice of method for summarising and displaying the data. For example, we showed that, when data contain outliers, the more *robust* or *resistant* median is a more sensible measure of average than the mean, and the semi-interquartile range a better indication of spread than standard deviation.

Chapter 4 discussed various methods of comparing groups of data. In the first two examples – *Hint, hint* (see page 44) and *A question of taste* (see page 46) – we see that the dependent variables take the form of categories; that is, success/failure, and favourite psychology module. The appropriate method for summarising these nominal variables is to cross-tabulate the frequency or percentage of each response against the independent variable (hint/no hint, and Arts/Science). The resulting contingency tables clearly show the extent to which responses are associated with (or *contingent* upon) the independent variable. So, in determining how data should be summarised, the property of the dependent variable is an important consideration.

The remaining examples in Chapter 4 used data in the form of numbers, rather than categories. We saw data displayed in terms of averages and spread. Importantly, these examples also illustrated how the *design* of a study determines the best methods of organising and displaying results. Thus, in the independent groups example (*Quick on the draw*), the *overall* averages and variabilities of the two groups provide the basis for summarising the data. On the other hand, in the repeated measures example (*Coffee time*), data are compared in terms of the *change* or difference in each individual's performance between the two conditions and the variability of these difference scores.

BEFORE READING ON . . .

Look over the examples in Chapter 4. If necessary, re-read the comments above until you are satisfied that you understand the issues.

. . . now read on

Taking Chapters 4 and 5 together, you can see that, not only is the choice of method for organising data influenced by the properties of the dependent variable and the experimental design, but also by the *question* to be asked of the data. Compare the *Coffee time* example at the end of Chapter 4 with any of the examples in Chapter 5. All these examples may be described as repeated measures design, in so far as the same participants are tested under two conditions. So, how does the *Coffee time* example differ from the others?

Student: Is it because the independent variable in Coffee time *is controlled by the experimenter, while all the others are subject variables?*

Lecturer: No, but I can see what you're driving at. In any case, in the Consistency *example in Chapter 5, the two computer altitude tests were chosen, or controlled, by the experimenter.*

Student: Ah, I missed that. I'm afraid I'm stumped.

Lecturer: Well, what do we want to know in the Coffee time *example?*

Student: Whether there is a difference in each participant's performance between the two treatments – coffee *and* no coffee.

Lecturer: Good. Now look at the examples in Chapter 5. What are we interested in this time?

Student: Ah, right, in all the examples there are two measures, and we want to know if participants who score highly on one measure also score highly on the other, and vice versa. Or, in some cases, like the Party time *example, we*

want to know if those who score high on one measure score correspondingly low on the other measure, and vice versa.

Lecturer: Correct – if a little long-winded. Can you put it more succinctly?

Student: Um . . . we want to know if there is a relationship between the two variables.

Lecturer: Good. So you see, this time, it's not just the design of the study that determines how we should examine the data, though that is important, but the question we are asking. Often the distinction is fairly clear, but not always. For example, in the Height and weight *example, it makes no sense to ask whether people's heights differ from their weights – the only sensible question is whether they are related.*

Student: Ah, but in the Critical thinking *example, it makes sense to ask if A's and B's judgements are related and if they are different.*

Lecturer: That's why you need to keep your wits about you.

continued

Student: Also, in the Coffee time *example, are we not actually asking if there is a relationship between coffee-drinking and reaction time?*

Lecturer: Indeed. Remember that the term 'relationship' can be ambiguous. Think of it this way – in the Coffee time *example, we are interested in a relationship between the independent variable – with only two levels, remember – and the dependent variable, reaction time. We examine this relationship by* comparing *performance* across the two conditions. In the other examples, we are also interested in relationships, but this time between two measures, such as height and weight.

Student: Ah, so in the Chapter 5 examples there are no independent variables as such, unlike the Coffee time study.

Lecturer: Just so – such studies are known as **correlational designs**.

SUMMING UP: CHOOSING THE RIGHT TEST

Salesman: Good day Madam, can I be of assistance?

Client: I'd like to buy a statistical test, but I'm having trouble making up my mind.

Salesman: I see. Perhaps I can be of some help.

What sort of scores do you have? (Reaction times)

What question do you wish to. . . .

We hope you have been persuaded that choosing the appropriate statistical test is much more straightforward than you might at first have thought. Remember, it's a bit like buying a car – more straightforward than that, maybe! Just ask yourself a few basic questions. Figure 9.10 presents a schematic representation of the various statistical tests you have encountered so far. We recommend that you keep this flow chart handy and, as you encounter a test, use it to see where that test fits into the overall scheme. For convenience, the diagram is reprinted on the **front inside cover** of the book.

As well as showing you the statistical landscape, the flow chart also helps you decide what statistical methods to use, and when. Simply begin at the top and work your way down. Note the three main branching points, shown as three 'layers' in the diagram.

1. What type of scores do I have?

The big issue at this point is whether your dependent variable is in the form of categories (that is, a *nominal* variable), or a numerical scale (that is, an ordinal, interval or ratio variable). If the data are nominal, then the appropriate statistical methods are crosstabulation and χ^2. You need go no further. On the other hand, if your scores are at least an ordinal scale, you need to ask two more questions.

2. What question do I want to answer?

This question relates to the last student/lecturer dialogue. Here, you are asking about the type of question posed in your hypothesis, the important choice being

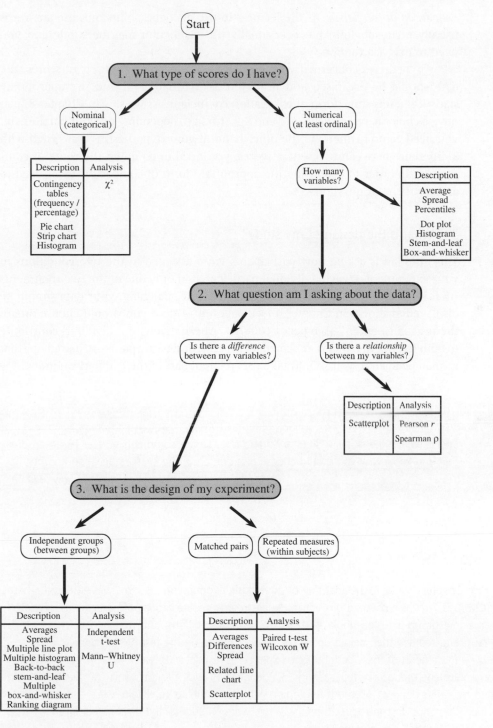

Figure 9.10 Decision chart

comparison or *correlation*. As the lecturer in the dialogue points out, the answer is usually pretty obvious, but occasionally the distinction may be subtle and you need to exercise caution.

For hypotheses concerned with a relationship between two sets of scores, the data should be organised and displayed as in Chapter 5, and the appropriate statistical test is some form of correlation coefficient. As we saw in Chapter 8, you have a choice between Pearson r and Spearman ρ, depending on your data. Again, you need go no further. On the other hand, if your hypothesis is concerned with a difference between two sets of scores, you need to go down the route of comparison. In order to determine the appropriate form of comparison, you need to answer the next question.

3. What is the design of my study?

This question is asking how participants were assigned to the two conditions in your experiment. If each individual participated in only one of the two treatments (that is, independent samples), and there was no matching, your data should be displayed as shown in Chapter 4 (see pages 50–3) and you should choose one of the tests in Chapter 7 (see pages 100–14). Alternatively, if individuals contribute to both treatments (that is, repeated measures), or if participants are paired up (that is, matched pairs), you should take the 'related' part of the comparison branch.

BEFORE READING ON . . .

Spend some time studying Figure 9.9 and refer to the comments above. Try to ensure that you know why you should choose one branch of the chart rather than another.

. . . now read on

CHAPTER REVIEW

Using examples from Chapters 4 and 7, the anatomy of three basic experimental designs was explored. These were independent groups, in which comparisons are made between separate groups of participants; repeated measures, where a single group is tested under both experimental conditions; and matched pairs, in which participants are first pre-tested and then paired up on the basis of matching pre-test performances.

The relative merits and demerits of these designs were explored in respect of threats to their internal validity, most notably non-equivalent groups (in the case of independent groups designs) and transfer effects (in relation to repeated measures designs). Methods for coping with these threats to validity were also discussed. Concepts of statistical inference, first introduced in Chapter 6, were extended, and level of significance, Type I and Type II errors, and statistical power were elaborated.

Finally, advice on how to choose the right statistical test was given, and a decision chart showing the relationship between the various tests was presented. For ease of access, this is repeated on the inside front cover.

Making sense of bigger designs

Seeing patterns in data: Comparing more than two groups

. . . we extend the methods of organising and displaying data to reveal patterns that were dealt with in Chapter 4. Whereas that chapter was restricted to comparisons between two groups of data, here we consider comparisons between more than two groups. By these methods, we can investigate empirically questions such as the following:

■ Do students from Arts, Science and Economics faculties differ in their attitudes to computers?

■ Do regular coffee and decaffeinated coffee affect speed of reaction relative to a (third) control condition?

The distinction, introduced in Chapter 4 and elaborated in Chapter 9, between three experimental designs, namely independent groups, repeated measures and matched pairs, is extended to comparisons between more than two groups.

EXAMPLES OF COMPARISONS

TECHNOPHILIA/TECHNOPHOBIA

Ways of measuring how people react to computers were discussed in Chapter 2 (see page 24). Figure 10.1 shows some real data collected from a class of first-year psychology students.

ARTS $N = 101$

54 47 44 56 53   41 61 56 52 58   43 50 55 58 53   53 54 46 44 48
54 54 57 47 54   52 56 55 52 48   48 43 39 56 55   54 67 51 45 61
52 55 41 47 47   43 61 47 57 59   60 43 54 66 52   67 44 59 52 50
44 50 58 54 50   68 56 45 58 52   42 67 57 45 47   50 46 56 56 44
52 53 45 51 49   34 58 59 60 56   54 61 61 59 49   45 53 50 60 44
41

SCIENCE $N = 39$

46 43 45 56 53   42 65 51 55 63   49 47 45 63 52   61 40 56 58 52
59 69 43 61 48   39 51 55 64 55   56 52 60 39 52   66 48 46 46

ECONOMICS $N = 33$

41 49 57 56 53   52 45 50 64 49   45 58 70 47 48   43 66 58 59 44
65 53 53 52 50   49 71 57 53 64   39 56 58

Figure 10.1 *Technophilia/technophobia* – computer attitudes for three faculties – real data

Summary statistics can be calculated for each of the faculties as follows:

	Arts	Science	Economics
Median	53	52	53
Semi-interquartile range	4.7	6.4	4.6
Mean	52.2	52.6	53.8
Standard deviation	6.8	8.0	8.1

BEFORE READING ON . . .

Study the table of summary statistics. What do they suggest?

. . . now read on

The most salient feature of the summary statistics is that they are very similar for all three faculties. Note also that the means and medians are extremely close together. (And remember the rule of thumb from Chapter 3, that standard deviation is likely to be roughly 1.5 times semi-interquartile range.)

The information on means and standard deviations is often shown graphically. In Figure 10.2 the points represent the means, and the lines stretch to 1 standard deviation above and below the mean in each case.

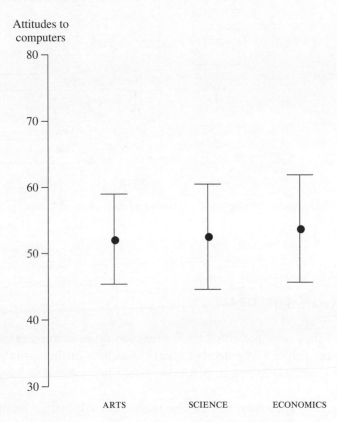

Figure 10.2 *Technophilia/technophobia* – standard deviations and mean computer attitude and standard deviation by faculty

The data can be summarized more fully using extensions of various graphical devices introduced in Chapter 4. Multiple histograms could be used, but are not particularly easy to interpret. Back-to-back stem-and-leaf plots obviously won't work for more than two groups. One of the best methods is to use multiple box-and-whisker plots. Figure 10.3 confirms the impression from the summary statistics – the distributions of attitutes to computer scores are very similar across the samples from the three faculties.

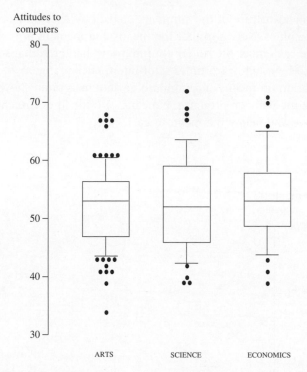

Figure 10.3 *Technophilia/technophobia* – box-and-whisker plots of computer attitude by faculty

QUICK ON THE DRAW

In Chapter 4 data were presented on the reaction times of samples of chess and squash players. Figure 10.4 extends the data to include further samples of bridge players and fencers. (Fencers, in particular, might be expected to have fast reaction times.)

Another graphical method that can be used effectively with a relatively small data set is *multiple line plots* (see Figure 10.5).

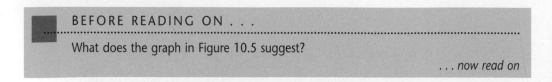

BEFORE READING ON . . .

What does the graph in Figure 10.5 suggest?

. . . now read on

It looks as if fencers and squash players have faster reaction times, with fencers somewhat faster on average. Chess and bridge players have longer reaction times, about the same overall.

SQUASH $N = 16$

27 32 34 41 31 30 32 37 33 30
35 32 38 29 28 23

CHESS $N = 15$

42 43 48 36 39 45 37 38 38 37
40 34 29 32 39

BRIDGE $N = 14$

35 38 33 46 29 34 49 35 41 36
37 37 43 31

FENCING $N = 15$

29 32 30 25 36 35 28 27 20 33
35 31 28 36 31

Figure 10.4 *Quick on the draw* – reaction times (centiseconds) for squash, chess, bridge and fencing

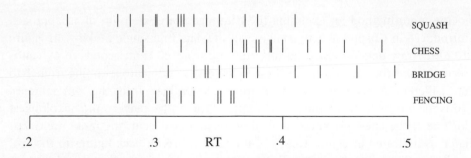

Figure 10.5 Multiple lire plots of squash, chess, bridge and fencing scores

BEFORE READING ON . . .

Use the line plots in Figure 10.5 to find the median for each group, and to estimate the semi-interquartile range, mean, and standard deviation (for the last, you can use the rule of thumb that about two-thirds of the data lie within 1 standard deviation above or below the mean). Use an appropriate software package to check the medians and your estimates of the other summary statistics.

. . . now read on

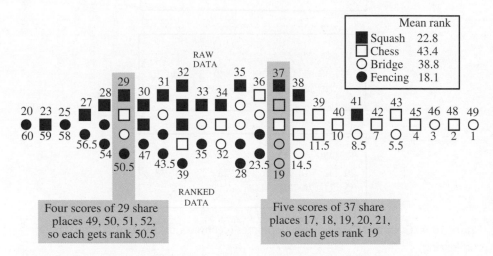

Figure 10.6 Combined ranking of squash, chess, bridge and fencing scores

One more method for exploring the data, again an extension of an approach introduced in Chapter 4, is to combine all the data in a single ranking. In Figure 10.6, the raw data are listed on top, running from 20 centiseconds to 49 centiseconds, and the ranks (from highest to lowest) underneath, running from 1 to 60. Different symbols are used to represent individuals from the four samples. Thus the longest reaction time was for one of the bridge players, the next longest for one of the chess players . . . and so on. When ties occur, the ranks are calculated as indicated in Figure 10.6. The preponderance of black figures to the left, and white figures to the right, reflects very clearly the pattern that squash players and fencers in the samples have faster reaction times than bridge and chess players.

COFFEE TIME

In Chapter 4, an example dealt with the effects of coffee on reaction time. In the experimental design described there, the same participants were tested under both

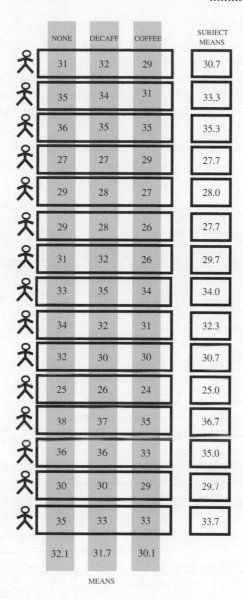

	NONE	DECAFF	COFFEE	SUBJECT MEANS
🚶	31	32	29	30.7
🚶	35	34	31	33.3
🚶	36	35	35	35.3
🚶	27	27	29	27.7
🚶	29	28	27	28.0
🚶	29	28	26	27.7
🚶	31	32	26	29.7
🚶	33	35	34	34.0
🚶	34	32	31	32.3
🚶	32	30	30	30.7
🚶	25	26	24	25.0
🚶	38	37	35	36.7
🚶	36	36	33	35.0
🚶	30	30	29	29.7
🚶	35	33	33	33.7
	32.1	31.7	30.1	
		MEANS		

Figure 10.7 *Coffee time* data – three repeated measures (RT csec.)

conditions – the control condition (without coffee) and the experimental condition (with coffee). This is an example of a *repeated measures design*. The design can be extended to more than two groups. Here we add another experimental condition – decaffeinated coffee, and the data to be considered are as shown in Figure 10.7.

The fact that this is a repeated measures design, so that each linked set of three data come from the same participant, is represented here by the stick figures in the diagram. The means for the three conditions, given at the bottom, show that, for this sample, reaction times were only slightly faster for the decaffeinated condition, but the coffee condition shows a larger effect of 2 centiseconds faster, on average. The mean for each participant can also be calculated, as indicated. These means can be used to compare participants for overall speed of reaction, and show that such speed varies considerably within the sample (or between participants) – from a mean of 25.0 to a mean of 36.7 – an aspect whose relevance will be considered later.

A ranking process can be carried out on the data. Here the three data for each participant are ranked (from highest to lowest) as indicated in Figure 10.8.

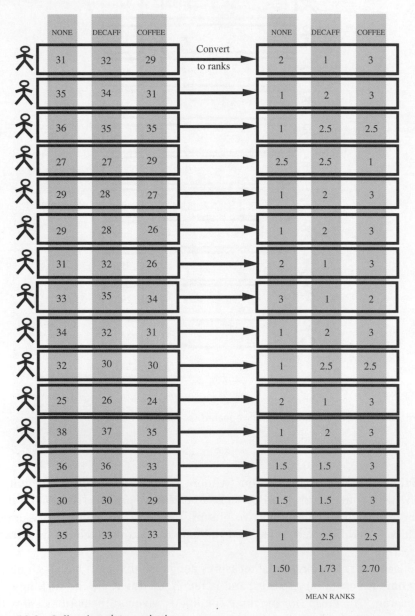

Figure 10.8 *Coffee time* data ranked

Having done this participant-by-participant ranking, the mean rank for each condition can be calculated. The mean rank for the decaffeinated condition is slightly higher than that for the control condition; but the mean rank for the coffee condition is considerably higher. The mostly salient pattern is that for the majority (13 out of 15) the reaction time is either lowest (that is, fastest) or equal lowest in the coffee condition, but there is relatively little difference overall for the control and decaffeinated conditions.

MAZE RUNNING

This example illustrates the third major type of experimental design, the *matched subjects design*. It concerns the effects of certain drugs, labelled A, B, and C, on the

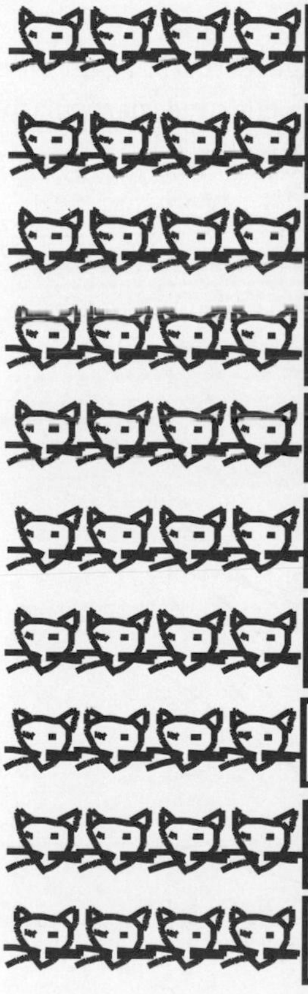

	CONTROL	A	B	C	LITTER MEANS
	48	43	49	57	49.3
	55	49	51	60	53.8
	62	52	53	62	56.8
	61	48	56	60	56.3
	45	47	43	46	45.3
	50	44	52	49	48.8
	51	51	47	54	50.8
	58	52	56	62	57.0
	69	62	68	70	67.3
	49	45	44	58	49.0
	54.8	49.3	51.9	57.8	

MEANS

Figure 10.9 *Maze-running* data (sec.) – 'matched rats' design

maze-running performance of mice (as measured by the number of seconds taken to get through the maze), relative to a control condition with no drug. If a repeated measures design were used – that is, each mouse ran the maze under each condition – there would be complications, since it is likely that the mouse's performance would improve with practice, or be subject to other order effects. As we saw in the previous chapter, there are ways to get round that difficulty in repeated measures designs, but here we consider a different approach – also discussed in Chapter 9. Mice are used in groups of four, with each group of four coming from the same litter. One member of each group of four is tested under each of the conditions. Because they come from the same litter, the mice within each group are related genetically and hence likely to be more similar in maze-running ability than mice from different litters, and this matching allows for a more controlled comparison between the experimental conditions. The data for the number of seconds taken to run the maze are shown in Figure 10.9.

It appears that, relative to the Control condition, drugs A and B enhance performance on the maze, leading to faster times on average, whereas drug D makes performance worse. Note also the wide variation in overall litter-by-litter performance.

The graphical method of showing the data as in Figure 10.10, again an extension of an approach introduced in Chapter 4, can be effective, particularly with

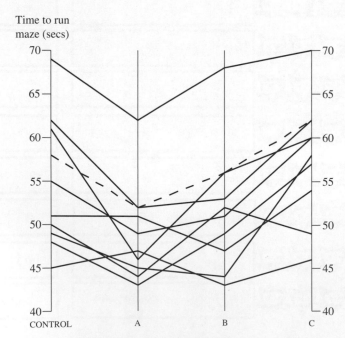

Note: one set of data plotted with dashed lines to avoid confusion because of overlap

Figure 10.10 Graphical display of *Maze-running* data

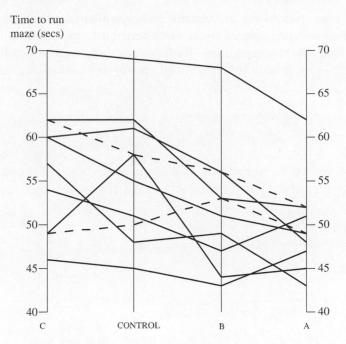

Figure 10.11 Rearranged graphical display of *Maze-running* data

smallish data sets. While Figure 10.10 shows the data clearly, in order to get the most from the graphical display it may be helpful to modify it slightly, as in Figure 10.11. Although precisely the same information is presented in both figures, note how the general trends within the data are more readily apparent from the rearranged display. As Figure 10.11 illustrates, in most cases the litter member treated with drug C took longer to run the maze than the undrugged litter member (seven out of ten cases, with one tie).

BEYOND GRAPHICAL ANALYSIS

The examples have illustrated how data may be displayed in forms that bring out the salient characteristics. Thus, from looking at the graphs, the data appear to provide some evidence that:

■ students in different faculties do not differ in their attitudes to computers;

■ squash players and fencers have faster reaction times than bridge and chess players;

■ decaffeinated coffee has no marked effect on reaction time but regular coffee does; and

■ Drugs A and B improve maze-running, but C makes it worse.

However, these conclusions are tentative. They are based on samples, whereas the questions we are interested in are more general. To provide a sharper analysis of the data, and the implications for the populations from which the samples are drawn, we need statistical tests, which are covered in the next chapter.

CHAPTER REVIEW

This chapter has extended graphical methods to comparisons involving more than two groups. Similarly, the distinction between three experimental designs – independent groups, repeated measures, and matched groups – generalises.

Statistical tests: Comparing more than two groups

IN THIS
CHAPTER
. . .

. . . we extend the tests covered in Chapter 7 to similar tests designed to compare more than two sets of data, building on the foundations laid in Chapter 10.

EXTENDING FROM TWO TO MORE THAN TWO GROUPS

As you saw in Chapter 7, for two independent groups, the independent (unpaired) t-test is a test of the null hypothesis that the samples come from populations with identical normal distributions. A rank-based alternative is the Mann–Whitney U test. For repeated measures or matched pairs designs, the paired (correlated) t-test is a test of the null hypothesis that the differences between pairs of data come from a population normally distributed with mean zero. The Wilcoxon Signed Ranks test is the corresponding rank-based test.

To show how all of these tests can be extended beyond two groups of data, we begin with two simple examples.

BEFORE READING ON . . .

The above is a fairly dense summary of the ideas in Chapter 7 concerning the comparison of unpaired and paired data sets, including the appropriate null hypotheses and rank-based alternatives. If you feel the need to refresh your memory of any of these ideas, now is the time to do so. Before continuing with this chapter, you should grasp the difference in approach between the unpaired and paired t-tests, particularly in respect of the null hypotheses, and the reasons for this.

. . . now read on

EXAMPLE 1: INDEPENDENT GROUPS

GENERAL KNOWLEDGE

For the purposes of explaining the general approach to comparing more than two independent groups, simple data have been made up for this example. To give an imaginable context, the 'cover story' is that samples of French, Irish and American students have been given a list of thirty-five capital cities – Rome, Paris, Dublin and so on – and asked to identify the corresponding countries. The data are their totals correct. To keep the example simple, the numbers are small (only eight in each sample) – much smaller than a serious study of this nature would use. Further, for simplicity, the numbers have been arranged so that the means come out as whole numbers. Moreover, to enable some important points to be made, we have presented two contrasting versions of data, as shown in Figure 11.1.

FRENCH	IRISH	US
22	21	16
18	25	20
21	27	18
23	25	18
19	23	15
19	20	14
24	26	19
22	25	16
21	24	17
	Means	

FRENCH	IRISH	US
16	23	18
27	28	14
26	16	25
19	27	27
14	18	11
25	31	12
26	26	15
15	23	14
21	24	17
	Means	

FIRST DATA SET SECOND DATA SET

Figure 11.1 *General knowledge* scores – contrasting data sets

Note that the means are the same for the two sets of data. Accordingly, if we tried to evaluate the evidence from these data for a difference in knowledge of world capitals among French, Irish and American students *only* on the basis of the differences between means in the samples, both data sets would lead us to the same conclusion. Yet, if we display the data graphically, a difference becomes obvious.

Looking at the first data set in Figure 11.2, the scores for the American students look quite different from the other two samples, but in the second data set, there

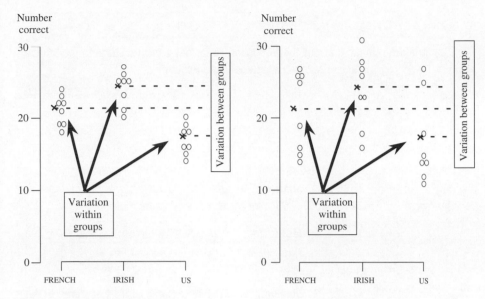

Figure 11.2 Graphs of *General knowledge* data

is considerably more overlap, and the difference is much less obvious. The under-lying distinction between the two data sets is that the data within each sample are much more spread out in the second data set than in the first. Just as with the independent t-test, it is necessary to take into account, not just the variation *between* groups – reflected in the differences between the group means – but also the variation *within* groups; that is, how spread out the data are within each of the groups.

A statistical approach called **Analysis of Variance** (**ANOVA** for short, pro-nounced 'ann-oh-vah') uses this basic idea – the relationship of variation between groups to variation within groups. In fact, ANOVA is a generalisation or exten-sion of the t-test.

Student: I'm a bit confused. You say this test called 'analysis of variance' can be thought of as a generalisa-tion of the t-test?

Statistician: That's right, the t-test is limited to cases where there are two sets of data to be compared, while ANOVA can be used to compare more than two sets.

Student: But the t-test analyses the difference between means of two data sets, whereas ANOVA analyses variation.

Statistician: Ah, I see where you're coming from. In fact, ANOVA does analyse the differences between the means of sets of scores.

Student: Then why is it called analysis of variance? Why not analysis of means, or analysis of differences?

Statistician: I suppose it could be, but analysis of vari-ance is a pretty good description of what the test, or more precisely the 'family' of tests, does.

Student: I've still not fully got my head around it. Why is it called analysis of variance?

Statistician: OK, but you already know the answer – you just haven't made the connection. Let's think about an independent t-test for a moment. Do you remember the basic rationale of that test?

Student: I think so. Basically, you calculate the difference between the two means and you divide it by some measure of the overall variability in the data. The bigger the difference in means compared to the variability, the bigger the t value and the more significant the difference. The larger the overall variability in the data compared to the difference between the means, the smaller the t value.

Statistician: That's pretty good. Now think about three sets of data. How would you calculate the difference between these means?

Student: Well, this time you have to compare three means, so you would subtract the first two, then subtract the second and third, then maybe subtract the first and third. But I'm not sure how you would summarise these three differences.

Statistician: Right, it could get pretty cumbersome. Imagine what you would have to do if there were five or six data sets or more.

Student: So, what we need is a single overall measure of the differences between all the means.

Statistician: Right again, you're nearly there. Now, can you think of a measure that corresponds to the differences between several scores?

Student: Ah, I think I see now – if a set of scores, in this case three means, differs a lot, we would say that they vary a lot.

Statistician: Correct! So a good way of expressing the differences between three or more means is to use a measure of variation.

Student: Something akin to variance, for example.

Statistician: See, I said you already knew the answer.

Student: So, in the case of a t-test, the difference between the two means can also be thought of as the variation between the two groups?

Statistician: That's certainly one way of thinking about it.

Student: So, can you do an ANOVA on just two sets of data instead of a t-test?

Statistician: Absolutely.

To return to our example: again, in keeping with our approach throughout this book, we do not present a calculation of ANOVA. Our expectation is that you will have access to software that will do the analysis for you. If an ANOVA is carried out for the first data set in our example, the ANOVA summary table will appear as in Figure 11.3.

SOURCE OF VARIATION	df	SUM OF SQUARES	MEAN SQUARE	F	p
Groups	2	197.333	98.667	19.923	.0000
Error	21	104.000	4.952		
Total	23	301.333			

Figure 11.3 *General knowledge* – ANOVA summary table for first data set

Source of Variation lists the systematic and non-systematic sources of variation discussed previously. The former is often referred to as *between* groups (here denoted by 'Groups') and the latter *within* groups, here labelled 'Error'. Why 'error' precisely? For complex historical reasons, this is the term that has been adopted conventionally, though the rationale for its use is by no means clear. We have simply to ask you to accept it as a piece of conventional terminology. A useful way to think about it is that it represents the unsystematic variation, attributable to individual differences within the population and other random influences, that remains after the systematic sources of variation have been taken out (here the only systematic source is differences between groups).

Sum of Squares (or **SS**) is a particular measure of variation for each source of variation, in the first case, the systematic variation between groups, in the second, error variation (in the sense explained above). As its name suggests, the SS (Total), which represents the overall variation in the data, is equal to the sum of the SS (Groups) and SS (Error). In other words, the entire variability in the data is explained by one or other of these sources of variation.

df stands for *Degrees of Freedom*, as usual. Again, a technical understanding of this term is beyond what we aim to cover in this book. Suffice it to say, for each calculation (in this case the Sums of Squares) the corresponding degrees of freedom correspond roughly, but not exactly, to the number of data points involved in that calculation (to be precise, the number of data points minus one, in this case). So, since 3 group means are used to calculate SS (Groups), the corresponding df is 3 − 1 = 2. Using precisely the same reasoning for SS (Total), the corresponding df is 24 − 1 = 23. The df for Error is calculated indirectly, that is, whatever is left over from the total Degrees of Freedom when the systematic dfs have been allocated – here there is only df (Groups) – hence, df (Error) = 23 − 2 = 21.

Mean Square (or **MS**) is a modified measure of variation found by dividing each Sum of Squares by its corresponding df. This helps to 'modulate' each measure of variation, since the SS (Group) is calculated using only three values, while SS for Error and Total use many more. So the latter two will tend to be larger simply by virtue of the fact that they were calculated using a greater number of scores to begin with.

F is the actual statistic for the test, as described above, that is, the ratio of the two Mean Squares (MS), in this case MS (Group) and MS (Error). Some points about the F statistic:

■ because of the way it is calculated, it is always positive;

■ the larger the value of F, the stronger the evidence from the data that there is a difference between the populations; and

■ as a rule of thumb, F needs to reach a value of approximately 4 to be statistically significant (the exact value depends on the dfs associated with the two Mean Squares).

p (or level of significance). The p value needs to be equal to or less than .05 for the result to be 'statistically significant at the .05 level'.

For the first data set in our example, you can see that F is large and the corresponding p value is very small – if fact, so small that it is .0000 rounded to 4 decimal places (this doesn't mean that it is zero – for example .00003 is .0000 if rounded off). These data indicate that the null hypothesis – that French, Irish and American students are equally knowledgeable about world capitals – can be rejected.

BEFORE READING ON . . .

Look again at the definitions of Source of Variation, Sum of Squares, Degrees of Freedom, Mean Square, F and p. It is important that you grasp the role that these elements play in Analysis of Variance. Although this is a relatively simple example, the ideas set out above generalise to all cases of ANOVA, regardless of how apparently complicated.
In order to consolidate your knowledge of the relationships between the various elements of the ANOVA summary table, fill in the blanks in Figure 11.4.

. . . now read on

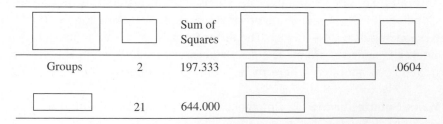

Figure 11.4 1-factor independent groups ANOVA – 'blank' summary table

Now let's consider the ANOVA summary table for the second data set (see Figure 11.5). You should recognise it as Figure 11.4. with the blanks filled in.

SOURCE OF VARIATION	df	SUM OF SQUARES	MEAN SQUARES	F	p
Groups	2	197.333	98.667	3.217	.0604
Error	21	644.000	30.667		

Figure 11.5 *General knowledge* – ANOVA summary table for second data set

---

BEFORE READING ON . . .

Compare the values in Figure 11.5 with your calculations. We hope they will tally – if not, check the calculations and try to figure out where you went wrong.

. . . now read on

Here you can see that the SS and MS for Groups are the same as for the first data set, reflecting the fact that the means are identical for both data sets. However, now the SS (Error) and MS (Error) are considerably bigger, reflecting the greater spread of data within the groups. As a consequence, the F ratio is much lower, and in fact, not high enough to reach statistical significance at the .05 level, as indicated by the p value of .0604 (greater than .05). If these data had been obtained in an experiment, therefore, the conclusion would have been to *fail to reject* the null hypothesis.

Student: *So, for the first data set, the ANOVA summary table tells us that the groups differ significantly in their knowledge of world capitals, but for the second data set, the groups don't differ significantly?*

Statistician: *Correct. More formally, we would say that there is a significant **main effect** of Groups for the first data set.*

Student: *And no significant main effect of Groups for the second set?*

Statistician: *Right, and remember, the means for the three groups were identical in each data set.*

Student: *But, in the first data set, the variability because of the systematic source of variance (that is, Groups), is sufficiently large compared to the variability of non-systematic sources (that is, Error), to allow us to reject the null hypothesis?*

Statistician: *Correct, but not so for the second data set.*

Student: *Done and dusted, as they say!*

Statistician: *Not so fast – we've not quite finished. Given that we have obtained a significant main effect of Groups, what can we conclude?*

Student: *Eh, that the three groups differ significantly from each other in their knowledge of world cities?*

continued

Statistician: *Possibly, but a significant main effect gives rise to several possibilities. All an ANOVA tells you is that, somewhere across the levels of your independent variable, there is a difference. It may be that all three means differ significantly. Equally, it may be that mean 1 differs from means 2 and 3, but the latter two don't differ from each other. Or means 2 and 3 may differ, but neither differ from mean 1, and so on.*

Student: *Oh, so just because you have a significant main effect, you can't assume that all your means differ significantly?*

Statistician: *Correct, you have to do more digging to identify the precise nature of the differences.*

Student: *How do you do that then?*

Statistician: *The process of digging around is known as* post hoc *testing. We shall come back to this later.*

EXAMPLE 2: REPEATED MEASURES

FADING MEMORIES

Again, we shall use some fictitious, simplified data to show how to analyse more than two groups where the data are linked – either because a *repeated measures design* has been used (for example, *Coffee time* on page 180 in Chapter 10) or a *matched groups design* (for example, *Maze-running* on page 183 in Chapter 10). The cover story is that eight participants learn a list of thirty words, and each individual is tested three times for recall of these words – 1 day, 2 days and 3 days later, giving data as shown in Figure 11.6.

BEFORE READING ON . . .

Spend some time considering the data in Figure 11.6. Can you detect any additional systematic source of variation (or information) that was not available in the previous example? (Hint: Note the contrast between the design of this example and the previous one.)

. . . now read on

How did you do? We hope you managed to distinguish *three* sources of variation in this example – two systematic and one non-systematic. There is, of course, the variation *between conditions*, reflected in the means – 17 for 1 day; 15 for 2 days; 10 for 3 days. However, in contrast to the previous example, we can also 'track' individual participants across the three conditions and look at their changes in performance. This gives us an additional systematic source of variation, called

	Original data				PARTICIPANT		Relative to means		
	DAYS				MEANS		DAYS		
	1	2	3				1	2	3
P1	24	22	14		20		4	2	–6
P2	13	14	6		11		2	3	–5
P3	17	12	10		13		4	–1	–3
P4	12	15	9		12		0	3	–3
P5	20	18	13		17		3	1	–4
P6	19	17	12		16		3	1	–4
P7	19	14	9		14		5	0	–5
P8	12	8	7		9		3	–1	–2

Figure 11.6 *Fading memories* data – three repeated measures

between subjects variation. *(Note: In keeping with current thinking, where possible, we prefer to use the term 'participant' rather than 'subject'. However, to avoid undue confusion, we continue to use 'subject' when it is intended as a technical term.)*

We can calculate a mean of the three scores for each participant as indicated, which constitutes a baseline for that individual. The overall variation in these means is essentially a measure of the magnitude of individual differences in reaction time among the sample. Each participant's data can then be recalculated relative to his/her mean, with the results shown (see also Figure 11.7). As in the previous example, the third source of variation is, of course, *Error*. In this case, the error variation is the variation in the *relative* scores. Now the ANOVA summary table appears as in Figure 11.8.

BEFORE READING ON . . .

Look back at Figure 11.3 the previous example for Independent Groups. Spend some time comparing the two summary tables and reflecting on the similarities and differences between them.

. . . now read on

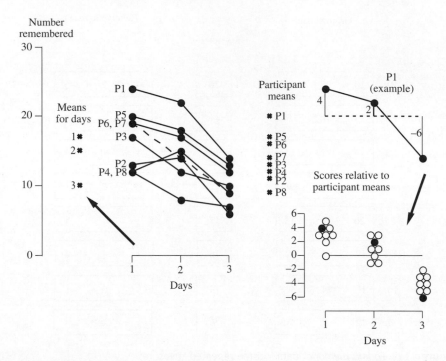

Figure 11.7 *Fading memories* – graphs of original recall scores and participants' recall relative to their baselines

SOURCE OF VARIATION	df	SUM OF SQUARES	MEAN SQUARE	F	p
Subjects		264.000			
Days	2	208.000	104.000	31.652	.0000
Error	14	46.000	3.286		

Figure 11.8 ANOVA summary table for *Fading memories* example

You will have noticed an extra line in Figure 11.8. This is to take account of the systematic differences *between subjects*. An F ratio is not calculated for this additional systematic source of variation, since it would only tell you whether there were overall differences between participants, which would not be particularly earth shattering. The F ratio for our independent variable is found by dividing the Mean Square for Days by the Mean Square for Error. For these data, F is statistically significant, as can be seen, indicating a significant main effect of Days.

ANOVA TERMINOLOGY

Some further terminology needs to be introduced at this point. In ANOVA, independent variables are referred to as **factors**. In this chapter, we are concerned only with ANOVA involving a single factor; that is, **one-factor** or **one-way** ANOVA. Chapter 13 deals with designs involving more than one factor. The different values that the factor can take are called **levels**. If an independent groups design is used, it is called a **between-groups** factor (since comparisons *between* separate groups are being made). If a repeated measures or matched groups design is used, it is called a **within-subjects** factor (since comparisons are being made *within* the same subjects, or *within* members of matched groups).

HEALTH WARNING!

Understandably, you may find the use of 'between' and 'within' terminology a little confusing here, since you have already encountered it in the context of between and within sources of variance. Bear in mind that, while there is a high degree of conceptual overlap between the two, one context does not map fully on to the other, so don't be tempted to think of them as meaning the same thing. Simply make sure you are aware of whether you are using the terms to identify sources of variation in your ANOVA, or whether you are using them to describe your factor.

ANOVA LOGIC: A SUMMARY

Having carried out an experiment involving one factor with three or more groups or treatments, we analyse the data for evidence of differences between the groups or treatments:

■ self-evidently, the data we obtain will not all be the same – the numbers *vary*;

■ some of this variation results from natural, *non-systematic* (random) sources;

■ some is caused by *systematic* differences in our data because of the independent variable (or factor);

■ ANOVA allows us to assess the relative amounts of variation attributable to non-systematic sources (or 'error') and to our independent variable (or factor);

■ this is done by computing an **F ratio**; that is, *taking a measure of the variation resulting from our factor and dividing by a measure of the variation caused by error*;

■ clearly, if our F ratio is *greater than 1*, the variation caused by the independent variable *outweighs* that caused by 'error';

■ if the F is *less than 1*, the variation resulting from the independent variable is *outweighed by* that caused by 'error';

■ the larger the value of F, the stronger the evidence from our data that there is a difference between the levels of our factor;

■ our judgement as to whether or not we can reject the null hypothesis will depend on *how much greater than 1* is the F ratio;

■ as a rule of thumb, F needs to reach a value of approximately 4 to be statistically significant (although the *exact* value of F for significance depends on the degrees of freedom);

■ the computer will calculate the F ratio and the corresponding p value; that is, the precise level of statistical significance;

■ by convention, the result of any analysis of variance is presented in an *ANOVA summary table* which is *always* organised under the following headings:

SOURCE OF VARIATION	df	SUM OF SQUARES	MEAN SQUARE	F	p

RANK-BASED ALTERNATIVES

As with all tests considered in this book, there are alternatives based on ranking procedures. These have, in fact, been anticipated in Chapter 10, and we pick up the examples again here.

REACTION TIMES – RANKED

Here again is the figure from Chapter 10 (see page 180) showing the combined data for reaction times of squash players, chess players, bridge players and fencers (see Figure 11.9). There is one difference, however – in Chapter 10 they were ranked 1–60 from highest to lowest. Here, instead, they have been ranked 1–60 from lowest to highest. Why? Simply because that is what computer programs do conventionally. (Note that when the order of ranking is reversed, a convenient way of calculating the new ranking in each case is to subtract the old rank from 61 – try it.)

For each of the four groups, the mean rank can be calculated as indicated. These means differ quite a bit, reflecting in particular that reaction times for squash players and fencers are generally faster than those for chess and bridge players, as was discussed earlier.

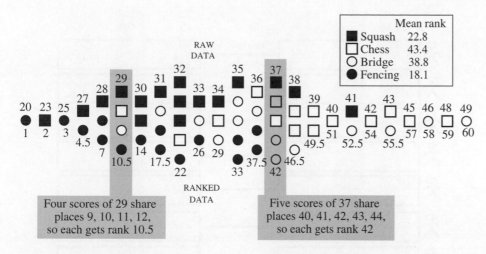

Figure 11.9 *Quick on the draw* – combined ranking of squash, chess, bridge and fencing scores

To test whether these differences in mean ranks are statistically significant, a test called the **Kruskal–Wallis** One Way ANOVA is used (you've guessed it, devised by statisticians Kruskal (William) and Wallis (Allen)). In line with our general philosophy, we expect you to use software to determine the value of the statistic associated with the test, and whether or not it is high enough to reach statistical significance. In fact, the appropriate statistic is distributed as the chi-squared statistic, with degrees of freedom 1 less than the number of groups (so 3 in this case). For our example, the result is:

$$\text{chi-square} = 22.2 \; df = 3 \; p = .0001$$

COFFEE TIMES – RANKED

Here again is the figure from Chapter 10 (see page 182) showing the reaction times under three conditions ranked participant-by-participant (see Figure 11.10). Again, the difference is that the order of rankings has been reversed to go from lowest to highest, because of computer software conventions. The mean ranks for the three conditions differ considerably – in particular, there is a marked tendency for the coffee condition to produce the lowest reaction time.

To test whether these differences are marked enough to reach the criterion of statistical significance, the appropriate test is called the **Friedman** test (yes, developed by economist Milton Friedman). Again, it results in a statistic that has the chi-square distribution (with degrees of freedom 1 less than the number of conditions), the result for this example being:

$$\text{chi-square} = 13.0 \; df = 2 \; p = .0015$$

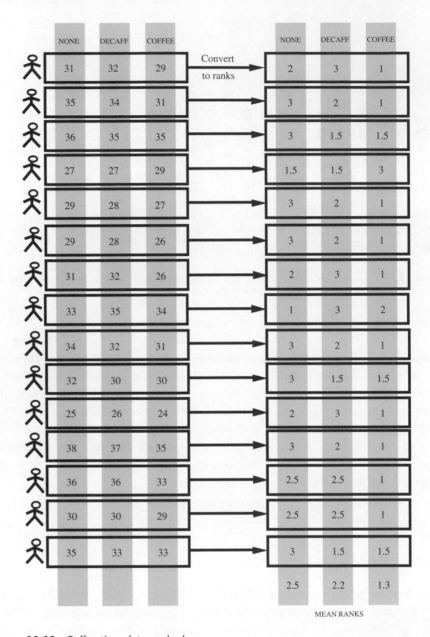

Figure 11.10 *Coffee time* data ranked

WHEN TO USE THE RANK-BASED ALTERNATIVES

There are no hard-and-fast rules as to when the rank-based alternatives are preferable to one-factor ANOVA. They are resistant to the effects of outliers, so one indication that they may be better is the existence in the data of prominent outliers – but there are no firm guidelines on exactly how outlying the outliers need to be to trigger the use of the rank-based alternatives. They are also preferable if there is an indication, either from the distribution of the samples, or on general grounds, that the distribution of the dependent variable in the population departs markedly from the normal distribution.

There are other, more obvious, circumstances where the rank-based tests are the only possible ones to use; namely, when the original data are themselves ranks. One example of each type will serve to illustrate this point.

A possible scenario is that you want to compare the mathematics performance of three groups of children within a class – those with a computer at home, those with a calculator, and those with neither – and that the data on mathematics performance available to you is a ranking by the teacher of all the pupils in the class. Then a Kruskal–Wallis test would be appropriate. (It must be said that these circumstances – where a lot of people are ranked on some variable, rather than measured in some way – are not likely to occur very often.)

It is more common for repeated measures to take the form of rankings, in particular when a number of objects are rated by a several individuals. For example, students might be asked to rank four psychology courses – Psycholinguistics, Social Psychology, Statistics, Human–Computer Interaction – from most liked (1) to least liked (4). A Friedman test would be the appropriate way to analyse such data.

SETTLING DIFFERENCES: POST-HOC TESTS

As the last student/statistician dialogue revealed, an F ratio that reaches statistical significance allows us to say that the null hypothesis can be rejected. This implies *some* difference between the groups (for a between-factor ANOVA) or the conditions (for a within-factors ANOVA). However, it does not pinpoint the *precise* difference or differences, and a follow-up test is necessary to do that. (Note that this complication does not arise with t-tests – if you think about it, you will realise why.)

MULTIPLE COMPARISONS

Consider the first of the two data sets from our *General knowledge* example again, with the data shown graphically in Figure 11.11. The ANOVA summary table (Figure 11.3) shows a statistically significant F ratio for *Groups*, pointing to a difference between French, Irish and American students. However, there are three specific comparisons underlying our significant result:

French v. Irish;
French v. American; and
Irish v. American.
Which of these is statistically significant?

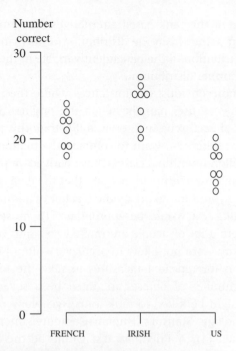

Figure 11.11 *General knowledge* – graph of first data set

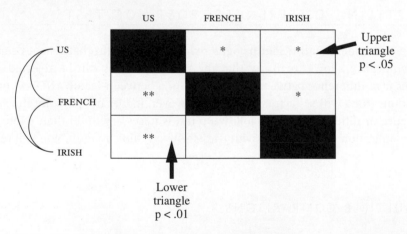

Figure 11.12 Results of Tukey's HSD tests (*General knowledge*)

A range of different methods is available for these comparisons, but we shall consider just one, which goes by the catchy title of **Tukey's Honestly Significant Difference (HSD) test**. Applying this test to our data using a standard computer package produces a summary of so-called *paired comparisons*. While the form of presentation may vary from one statistical package to another, each will present the same information, namely a summary of comparisons of all possible pairs of means. Figure 11.12 presents a format used frequently for summarising paired comparisons. The table has three features: (i) a *leading diagonal* (the black squares);

(ii) an upper triangle; and (iii) a lower triangle. The leading diagonal is entirely redundant, since it represents the comparison of each mean with itself. The upper and lower triangles are mirror images that represent identical comparisons, so, rather than present redundant information, it is possible to use each triangle to present the same comparisons at, say, different levels of significance.

In this case, the table shows which comparisons are statistically significant at the .05 level (upper triangle) and also at the more stringent .01 level. In our example, all three comparisons are statistically significant at the .05 level (as indicated by *). In fact, the differences between the French and US, and Irish and US students are statistically significant at the .01 level. (The curved lines on the left in the figure summarise which differences are significant at the .05 level; in this case, all of them.) Similarly, applying the same test to the control group/decaff/ coffee data produces the table shown in Figure 11.13.

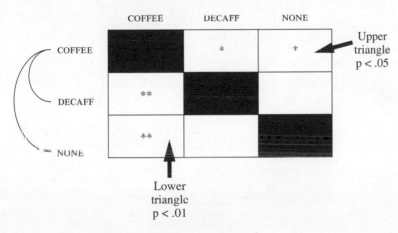

Figure 11.13   Results of Tukey's HSD tests (*Coffee time*)

BEFORE READING ON . . .

Interpret the table in Figure 11.13.

. . . now read on

TREND-SETTING

The levels of a factor in ANOVA often are values of a category variable – for example, faculty, nationality or experimental treatment. Since the ordering of the levels is arbitrary in these cases, it is sufficient to use multiple comparisons to discover what differs from what.

In some cases, however, the levels of a factor may have a natural order. A clear example is the memory experiment, in which the levels are the number of days elapsed (1, 2 or 3) since the items were committed to memory. In such cases, we are usually interested in more than merely whether one level of a factor differs from any other. Instead, we may wish to know whether there is a general **trend** across the levels of our factor.

As might be expected, the graphical analysis of the memory data does show a clear trend – the longer the time, the more forgetting takes place (Figure 11.14). Indeed, the data can roughly be fitted by a straight line, as indicated. In such a case, the variation associated with the experimental condition can be split into the variation relating to this linear trend, and the rest. In terms of the ANOVA summary table, this may be indicated as shown in Figure 11.15. The linear trend

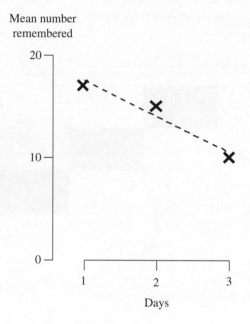

Figure 11.14 *Fading memories – trend across days*

SOURCE OF VARIATION	df	SUM OF SQUARES	MEAN SQUARE	F	p
Subjects		264.000			
Days	2	208.000	104.000	31.652	.0000
Linear trend	1	196.000	196.000	59.625	.0000
Error	14	46.000	3.286		

Figure 11.15 *Fading memories – ANOVA summary table including linear trend test*

is associated with 1 df, and an F ratio can be calculated. In this case, it will be seen that the linear trend accounts for a high proportion of the variance in experimental conditions, and the corresponding F ratio is very high, confirming the impression of a strong linear trend given by the graph.

PRACTICE MAKES YOU-KNOW-WHAT

We strongly recommend that you use some of the data sets provided in Chapter 10 to reinforce your ability to carry out and interpret the tests covered here.

CHAPTER REVIEW

In this chapter, *one-factor* (also known as *one-way*) ANOVA has been introduced, together with rank-based alternative tests and follow-up (*post hoc*) tests to pinpoint the nature of any differences indicated by a statistically significant result. The relationships between the tests for two samples – either independent or related – and those for more than two samples are summarised in Figure 11.16.

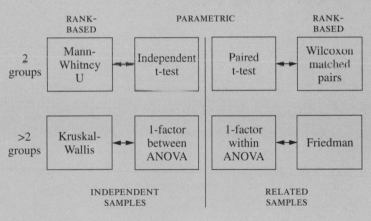

Figure 11.16 Relationships between tests

12 Seeing patterns in data: Comparisons involving more than one independent variable

...comparisons within more complex experimental designs are illustrated through summary statistics and graphs. Whereas Chapters 4 and 10 described comparisons based on a *single* independent variable with two or more levels, this chapter extends these ideas to comparisons involving *two* factors (independent variables). As in the earlier chapters, factors may be *between* (groups) or *within* (subjects), so there are three cases to be considered:

■ both factors between;

■ 1 between and 1 within factor; and

■ both factors within.

ILLUSTRATIVE EXAMPLES

TECHNOPHILIA/TECHNOPHOBIA

We have previously considered possible general differences between Faculties in terms of attitudes to computers. It might also be of interest to test whether there is any evidence of a gender difference. It would be possible to test this using a t-test for all the students together, or possibly three separate t-tests to compare females and males within each of the three faculties. However, a more powerful method is to consider Faculty and Gender together as two independent variables (or factors) within a single analysis.

In this example, there are two factors, namely Faculty and Gender. They are both *between* factors, since no student can belongs to more than one faculty or more than one gender. Faculty has three levels – Arts, Science and Economics; Gender has two levels – female and male.

Figure 12.1 displays the six combinations of two Genders by three Faculties. In each cell, the data are illustrated (not given in full), and the number of cases and mean are given for each cell. As well as these means, overall means can be worked out for:

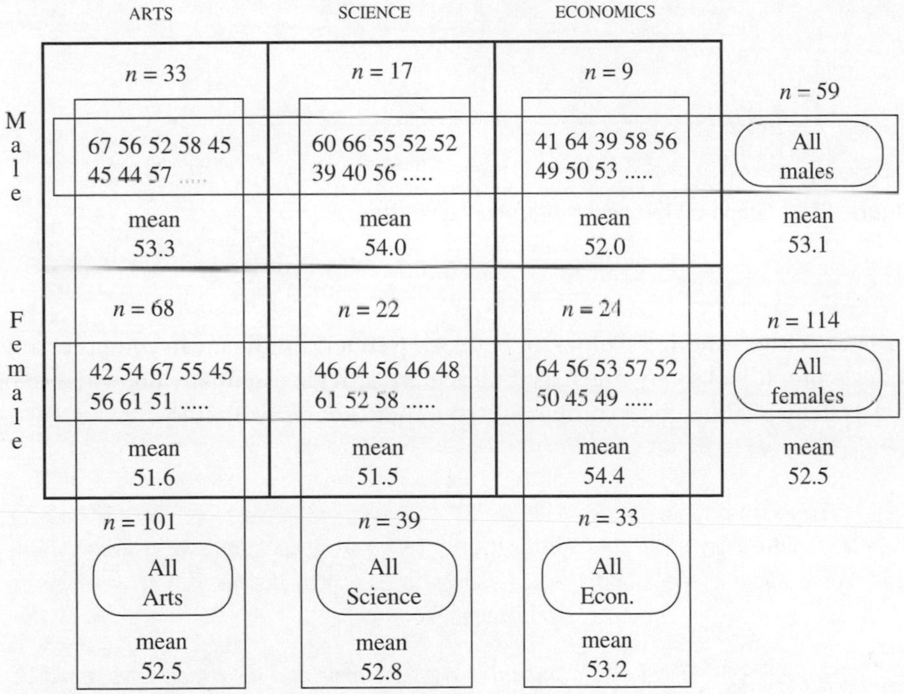

	ARTS	SCIENCE	ECONOMICS	
Male	$n = 33$	$n = 17$	$n = 9$	$n = 59$
	67 56 52 58 45 45 44 57	60 66 55 52 52 39 40 56	41 64 39 58 56 49 50 53	All males
	mean 53.3	mean 54.0	mean 52.0	mean 53.1
Female	$n = 68$	$n = 22$	$n = 24$	$n = 114$
	42 54 67 55 45 56 61 51	46 64 56 46 48 61 52 58	64 56 53 57 52 50 45 49	All females
	mean 51.6	mean 51.5	mean 54.4	mean 52.5
	$n = 101$	$n = 39$	$n = 33$	
	All Arts	All Science	All Econ.	
	mean 52.5	mean 52.8	mean 53.2	

Figure 12.1 *Technophilia/technophobia* – computer attitudes by faculty and gender – partial data for illustration

■   all males, all females; or

■   all Arts students, all Science students, all Economics students, as indicated.

Having calculated the means for each Gender/Faculty combination, they can be displayed effectively using the sort of graph shown in Figure 12.2. From this graph (as from the original table showing means) it can be seen that there is very little

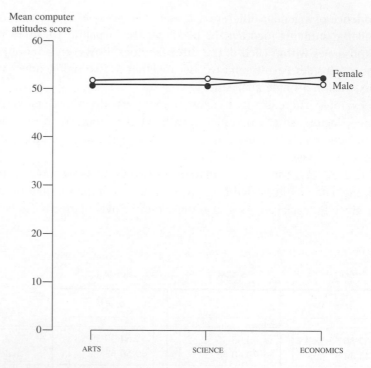

Figure 12.2 Graph of *Technophilia/technophobia* data

variation either among Faculties, or between Genders, in the mean computer attitudes score. It looks very much as if these data provide essentially no evidence of any systematic differences attributable to either Gender or Faculty.

Student: Why did you choose to put Faculty along the horizontal axis and have two separate lines for males and females within the graph?

Statistician: This was an entirely arbitrary decision. We could just as well have put Gender on the X-axis and embedded Faculty within the graph.

Student: How would I know which to do on any occasion?

Statistician: Often it doesn't matter, since both graphs convey identical information, so you will never be wrong. Sometimes, though, one representation may be more convenient for illustrating a point.

Student: What do you mean by that?

Statistician: Let's look at the graph we've drawn. How would you tell if there was a difference between males and females?

Student: Well, the male and the female lines would be quite distinct.

Statistician: That's right. So for the factor that we have 'embedded' in the graph, the vertical displacement of the lines will indicate the magnitude of the effect of that variable. Now what about the effect of Faculty?

Student: Ah, that would be shown by the lines sloping in one direction or the other. So for one factor, an effect is illustrated by how far apart the lines are, and for the other factor, the steepness of the lines?

Statistician: Correct, and sometimes an effect you are interested in may be more immediately apparent in one representation than the other. Often, it's a matter of preference and of trying out the different representations.

Student: So, depending on the data, a graph could show vertical displacement but no slope, slope but no vertical displacement, and both or neither.

Statistician: Yes, and more complicated patterns besides as we'll see below.

COUCH POTATOES

Figure 12.3 shows some data on the average number of hours (to the nearest hour) children spent watching TV. The data are analysed in terms of the social class of the father, and the age of the child. For each combination of social class of father/age of child, data for six children are listed in the row. The mean for each group of six children is shown in the final column.

BEFORE READING ON . . .

How many factors are there in this study, and what type is each? How many levels are there of each factor?

. . . now read on

SOCIAL CLASS OF FATHER	AGE	HOURS TV PER WEEK	MEANS
AB	6	17 22 13 21 15 19	17.8
	10	21 19 15 18 22 14	18.2
	14	11 19 17 12 23 15	16.2
C1	6	25 14 18 20 18 18	18.8
	10	27 23 10 18 24 23	20.8
	14	17 22 15 21 26 19	20.0
C2	6	26 22 18 19 15 19	19.8
	10	19 25 29 14 25 16	21.3
	14	24 11 24 27 22 23	21.8
DE	6	19 16 28 23 17 24	21.2
	10	21 17 31 19 25 25	23.0
	14	13 35 26 21 17 22	22.3

Figure 12.3 *Couch potato data*

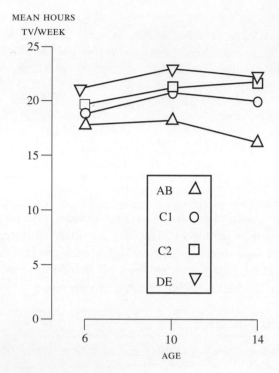

Figure 12.4 Graph of *Couch potato* data

Again, the simplest way to look at the patterns in the data is to graph the means as in Figure 12.4.

BEFORE READING ON . . .

What patterns do you see in this graph? Jot down your thoughts.

. . . now read on

The apparent patterns are:

■ a clear relationship between social class of father and amount of TV watching. As social class goes progressively from AB to DE the average amount of viewing consistently increases; and

■ not much indication of change with age – slightly lower figures for the 6-year-olds.

As an exercise, you might like to replot the graph with social class of father along the axis and a separate line for each of the three ages.

FADING MEMORIES

In this experiment, participants were asked to memorise a list of thirty words, and each participant was tested for the number correctly recalled 1 day, 2 days, 3 days and 4 days later. In addition, an experimental condition was included whereby half the participants were taught a mnemonic strategy beforehand (experimental group) and the other half were not (control group), with seven participants in each group. Data are presented in Figure 12.5.

| | | DAYS | | |
		1	2	3	4
NO STRATEGY TRAINING		20	13	8	5
		23	18	13	11
		19	15	12	7
		25	19	14	13
		20	17	16	11
		16	9	5	4
		24	15	11	7
MEANS		21.0	15.1	11.3	8.3
STRATEGY TRAINING		28	26	22	23
		24	21	20	20
		27	27	22	21
		27	23	21	19
		26	23	18	19
		22	20	19	20
		22	18	17	17
MEANS		25.1	22.6	19.9	19.9

Figure 12.5 *Fading memories*– recall scores by strategy and day

BEFORE READING ON . . .

Identify the factors and say which type each one is. How many levels for each factor?

. . . now read on

In this case there are two factors – experimental condition is a *between* factor with two levels, and number of days elapsed is a *within* factor with four levels (1, 2, 3, 4 days). This type of design is known formally as a **2-factor mixed design** (*mixed* because one factor is between and the other within). Plotting the means leads to the graph in Figure 12.6.

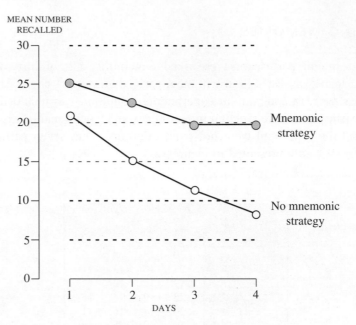

Figure 12.6 Graph of *Fading memories* data

It appears from the graph that:

■ memory deteriorates over the time period, *irrespective of the learning strategy* – this is called a *main effect* of Days;

■ the mnemonic strategy has a beneficial effect in aiding recall, *irrespective of the number of days* – this time a *main effect* of Strategy; and, moreover,

■ the rate of forgetting, as shown by the slope of the line, is less slow for the experimental group than for the control group.

When the pattern across one factor (here the *time elapsed*) differs for different levels of the other factor (*experimental* or *control*) this is called an **interaction**. In this example, then, it appears that there is an *interaction* between time elapsed and experimental condition – a **(Day × Strategy) interaction**, as well as a main effect for time elapsed and a main effect for experimental condition.

FAME AND RECOGNITION

In this experiment male and female students (eight of each) were shown 60 photographs – 20 of fashion models, 20 of footballers, and 20 of pop stars – and asked to identify them. The data are the number correct (see Figure 12.7). This is another example with 1 between factor and 1 within factor – a *2-factor mixed design*. Here the between factor is Gender (with two levels, as usual) and the within factor is Category of photograph (with three levels). If you look at the total scores out of 60, you can see from the table that the means for males (30.6) and females (30.9), *irrespective of category*, are essentially the same – we can express this by saying that there appears to be no main effect of Gender. Similarly, the overall means for the three categories, *irrespective of gender*, are very close (10.1, 10.3 and 10.3, respectively). So it might appear that there are no interesting effects in these data. That this would be a wrong conclusion is evident when the data are graphed, as in Figure 12.8 (you may have noticed it from the table).

Here there is a very strong **(Gender × Category) interaction**, even though

	MODELS	FOOTBALLERS	POP STARS	TOTAL
MALE	7	15	11	33
	4	12	5	21
	5	17	9	31
	11	18	14	43
	8	15	8	31
	8	16	13	37
	3	14	11	28
	4	16	6	26
MEANS	6.1	15.1	9.3	30.6
FEMALE	10	3	11	24
	17	10	14	41
	17	11	17	45
	15	5	11	31
	18	5	10	33
	11	4	9	24
	12	2	9	23
	15	7	12	34
	12	3	8	23
MEANS	14.1	5.6	11.2	30.9
OVERALL MEANS	10.1	10.3	10.3	

Figure 12.7 *Fame and recognition* – identification scores by gender and type of photograph

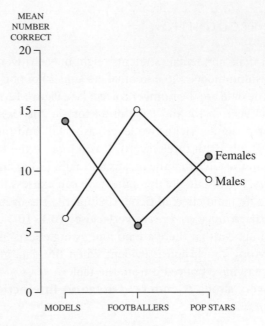

Figure 12.8 Graph of *Fame and recognition* data

neither factor produces a main effect. The interaction arises because the males are much better at identifying footballers, and females at identifying fashion models – in terms of the total scores, these differences balance out.

HOT AND BOTHERED

To complete the picture, here are some data from an experiment involving two within factors – a *2-factor repeated measures design*. Eight experienced typists are tested for their typing speed (words per minute) under three levels of noise (low, moderate, high) combined with three ambient temperatures (50°F, 55°F, 60°F), yielding nine combinations, as indicated in Figure 12.9. The graph in Figure 12.10 has temperature plotted on the horizontal axis and a separate line for each level of noise. (What if you plot level of noise on the horizontal axis and a separate line for each temperature? Is one arrangement better than the other?)

From the graph, it would appear that:

■ performance deteriorates as noise level increases, irrespective of temperature;

■ performance is better at 55°F than either colder or hotter, irrespective of noise level; and

■ the pattern across temperatures is the same for each level of noise, which we can express by saying that there is no sign of a *(Noise × Temperature) interaction*.

NOISE	LOW			MODERATE			HIGH		
TEMP.	50°	55°	60°	50°	55°	60°	50°	55°	60°
S1	90	94	89	85	90	87	77	85	77
S2	78	86	80	76	85	73	68	77	69
S3	88	90	89	82	88	87	80	80	83
S4	86	93	90	82	85	86	72	78	72
S5	76	84	76	75	80	71	66	72	66
S6	79	85	81	73	81	73	69	73	71
S7	83	90	85	78	84	79	71	80	71
S8	80	85	83	77	81	78	71	72	68
Means	82.5	88.4	84.1	78.5	84.3	79.3	71.8	77.1	72.1

Note: Temperature in degrees Fahrenheit

Figure 12.9 *Hot and bothered* – typing speed (wpm) by noise and temperature

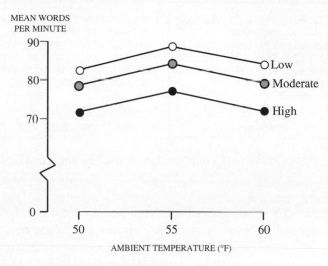

Figure 12.10 Graph of *Hot and bothered* data

PICTURES IN THE MIND

In a well-known experiment on perception, participants are presented with simple figures, such as the letter F, with the following variations as shown in Figure 12.11:

■ the figure is normal, or reversed; and/or

■ it is rotated through varying angles.

The task is to decide, as quickly as possible, if the letter is normal or reversed, and the dependent variable is the time (in milliseconds) to make this decision.

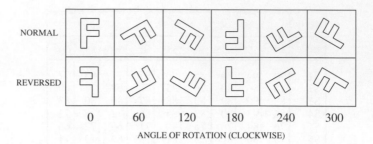

NORMAL

REVERSED

	0	60	120	180	240	300

ANGLE OF ROTATION (CLOCKWISE)

Figure 12.11 *Pictures in the mind* – six angles of rotation and two figure types (normal and reversed)

NORMAL						REVERSED					
ANGLE OF ROTATION (CLOCKWISE)						ANGLE OF ROTATION (CLOCKWISE)					
0	60	120	180	240	300	0	60	120	180	240	300
552	621	789	1067	780	630	609	670	835	1124	828	678
533	601	760	1048	771	598	579	648	812	1097	822	644
565	611	777	1061	773	615	615	666	828	1112	823	665
521	578	734	1021	740	584	566	631	789	1078	788	631
589	649	801	1091	798	646	638	697	852	1141	841	699
547	599	749	1027	752	607	599	644	796	1072	798	652
551	610	768	1053	769	613	601	659	819	1102	817	662
MEANS						MEANS					

Figure 12.12 *Pictures in the mind* – response time (msec.) by angle and type

If each participant is tested with all twelve variations, the design has two *within* factors, with two and six levels. Again, this is known as a *2-factor repeated measures design*. Figure 12.12 presents some representative data for such an experiment with six participants – the resultant graph is shown in Figure 12.13.

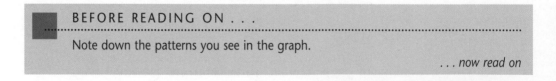

BEFORE READING ON . . .

Note down the patterns you see in the graph.

. . . now read on

Clearly, as the angle increases to 180°, the time to determine whether the figure is reversed or not increases. Thereafter it decreases, symmetrically. Since a clockwise rotation of 240° is equivalent to an anticlockwise rotation of 120°, and clockwise 300° is the same as anticlockwise 60°, this symmetry indicates that it is the size of the angle that determines the time, regardless of whether the rotation is

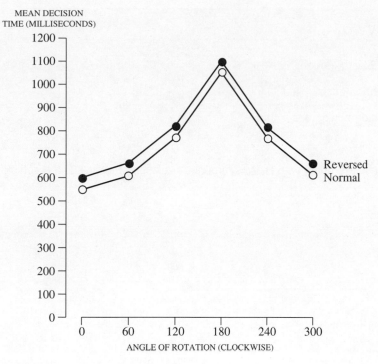

Figure 12.13 Graph of *Pictures in the mind* data

clockwise or anti-clockwise. So there is clearly a *main effect* for angle of rotation; that is *irrespective of the normal/reversed factor*. The data are consistent with an explanation that the decision as to whether the figure is reversed or not is made by first mentally rotating it (at constant speed) into its normal orientation and then checking whether the rotated image is normal or reversed.

Second, the reversed figures consistently take longer (by about 50 milliseconds) than the normal figures. This small increment in decision time for reversed figures is *irrespective of the angle of orientation*; that is, a *main effect* for the normal/reversed factor.

The pattern of response times for normal and reversed figures looks pretty independent of the angle of rotation (and vice versa), indicating *no interaction* between the two factors.

BEYOND GRAPHICAL ANALYSIS

In line with our approach, this chapter has introduced examples of data for 2-factor experimental designs. However, the graphical analysis of such data, while it may be indicative of patterns in the data, needs to be followed by statistical tests, and these are the subject for the next chapter.

CHAPTER REVIEW

In this chapter, three types of 2-factor design:

■   2 between (all independent groups);

■   1 between, 1 within (2-factor mixed); and

■   2 within (all repeated measures)

have each been illustrated by two examples, with analysis through calculation of means, and graphically.

Statistical tests: Comparing more than one independent variable

. . . the examples examined graphically in Chapter 12 are revisited, using Analysis of Variance (ANOVA) to test for which differences are statistically significant. Various follow-up tests designed to pinpoint more precisely the nature of statistical significance are also explained.

FOR EXAMPLE . . .

TECHNOPHILIA/TECHNOPHOBIA

Here, again, is the graph of the data introduced in Chapter 12 (page 208) for attitudes to computers among students in relation to Faculty and Gender (see Figure 13.1). This is an example of a **two-factor design**, with Faculty and Gender as our factors. Since there are two factors, the data are analysed using a version of ANOVA known as **two-factor**, or **two-way**, ANOVA. Moreover, since both factors are examples of unrelated, or *between groups*, variables, the analysis is a **two-way between (groups) ANOVA**. The summary table for this analysis is given in Figure 13.2.

Here, there are four sources of variation:

■ differences between faculties – reflected in the graph, and in the faculty means (very small differences, so variation is small);

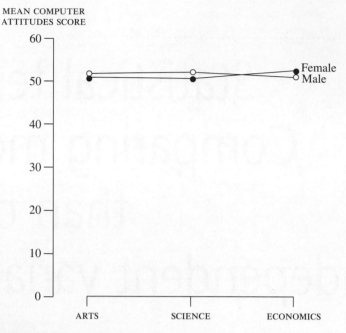

Figure 13.1 Graph of *Technophilia/technophobia* data

SOURCE OF VARIATION	df	SUM OF SQUARES	MEAN SQUARE	F	p
Faculty	2	11.089	5.545	.103	.9018
Gender	1	10.890	10.890	.203	.6528
FG interaction	2	138.924	69.462	1.295	.2765
Error	167	8954.946	53.622		

GENDER MEANS

Male	53.1
Female	52.5

FACULTY MEANS

Arts	52.5
Science	52.8
Economics	53.2

Figure 13.2 ANOVA summary table for *Technophilia/technophobia* example

■ differences between genders – reflected in the graph, and in the gender means (again, very small differences, so variation again small);

■ interaction between faculties and gender (no indication of an interaction in the graph); and

■ 'error' variation – the 'background variation' resuling simply from individual differences.

The first three are *systematic* sources of variation, while the fourth is *non-systematic*. Although this example may appear more complex than the one-factor ANOVAs discussed in Chapter 11, the basic approach is identical. For each of the three systematic sources of variation, an F ratio is obtained by dividing the Mean Square term in question by the MS (Error). As can be seen, each of these F ratios is small and, correspondingly, the p values are well above .05, so none of the three is statistically significant, confirming what the graph suggests strongly – that there is no indication from these data that attitudes to computers depends on either Faculty or Gender, or the interaction between these two factors.

BEFORE READING ON . . .

In order to help consolidate your knowledge of how F ratios are obtained, fill in the blanks in Figure 13.3. Bear in mind that the relationships between the various elements in the summary table are identical to the one-way case in Chapter 11, the only difference being that there are three systematic sources of variation, rather than one. You can check your calculations below.

. . . now read on

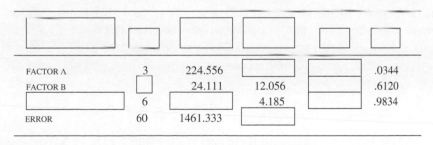

Figure 13.3 2-factor unrelated ANOVA – 'blank' summary table

COUCH POTATOES

Figure 13.4 presents a graph of the data on the amount of TV viewing by children of different ages, related to social class of father, this time plotted differently from before. Again, this example has *two between* factors.

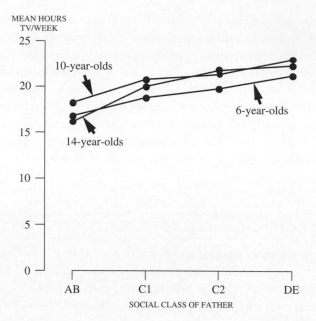

Figure 13.4 Graph of *Couch potato* data

BEFORE READING ON . . .

Look back at the corresponding graph in Chapter 12 (see page 210). Remember, both versions contain the same mean scores and convey identical information. Study these graphs and consider how each version allows you to view the same data from different perspectives. What effects are more apparent in each version?

. . . now read on

The ANOVA summary table for these data is shown in Figure 13.5. You should recognise it as Figure 13.3 with the blanks filled in.

BEFORE READING ON . . .

Compare the values in the summary table with your own. Check any calculations that do not tally.

. . . now read on

Here the F ratio for the *main effect* of social class of father (Class) does reach the level required to be statistically significant (the p value is just below .05). Neither the *main effect* for Age, nor the *interaction* between Class and Age, is statistically

SOURCE OF VARIATION	df	SUM OF SQUARES	MEAN SQUARE	F	p
Class	3	224.556	74.852	3.073	.0344
Age	2	24.111	12.056	.495	.6120
CA interaction	6	25.111	4.185	.172	.9834
Error	60	1461.333	24.356		

CLASS MEANS

AB	17.39
C1	19.89
C2	21.00
DE	22.17

AGE MEANS

6	19.42
10	20.83
14	20.08

Figure 13.5 ANOVA summary table for *Couch potato* example

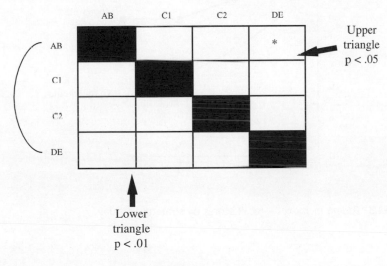

Figure 13.6 *Couch potato* – Tukey's HSD tests

significant. Applying Tukey's Honestly Significant Differences test produces the table shown in Figure 13.6. As can be seen, there is only one pairwise comparison that is statistically significant. However, in this case, what is more important than individual pairwise comparisons is the overall *trend*, which is very clear when the data are replotted with social class of father along the horizontal axis. A linear trend test adds another line to the ANOVA summary table, as seen in Figure 13.7. It can be seen that most of the variation caused by differences in social class of father is accounted for by the linear trend, and the F ratio for this trend is highly statistically significant.

SOURCE OF VARIATION	df	SUM OF SQUARES	MEAN SQUARE	F	p
Class	3	224.556	74.852	3.073	.0344
Linear trend	1	214.678	214.678	8.814	.0043
Age	2	24.111	12.056	.495	.6120
CA interaction	6	25.111	4.185	.172	.9834
Error	60	1461.333	24.356		

Figure 13.7 ANOVA summary table for *Couch potato* data, including linear trend test

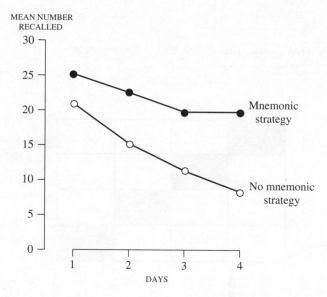

Figure 13.8 *Fading memories* – recall scores by strategy and day

Fading memories

Figure 13.8 again shows the graph for the experiment involving memory deterioration over time for an experimental group given training in a mnemonic strategy and a control group given no such training. By contrast with the first two examples, which involved two *between* factors, this is an example of a **mixed design**, with one between factor (experimental versus control group) and one within factor (days elapsed). The ANOVA summary table (including linear trend for days) is as shown in Figure 13.9.

Note that there are two error terms in this table, one for working out the F ratio for the main effect of the between factor, and the other for working out the F ratio for the main effect of the within factor, as well as that for the interaction. An explanation of why this is so will not be offered! Suffice it to say that the different error terms are a consequence of the fact that one factor is between and

SOURCE OF VARIATION	df	SUM OF SQUARES	MEAN SQUARE	F	p
Mnemonic	1	880.071	880.071	29.642	.0001
Error	12	356.286	29.690		
Days	3	668.358	222.786	118.443	.0000
Linear trend	1	642.057	642.057	341.347	.0000
MD interaction	3	98.929	32.976	17.532	.0000
Error	36	67.714	1.881		

MNEMONIC MEANS	
No training	13.93
Training	21.86

DAYS MEANS	
1 day	23.07
2 days	18.86
3 days	15.57
4 days	14.07

Figure 13.9 ANOVA summary table for *Fading memories* data, including linear trend test

the other within. In practice, it makes no difference whatever in the way you should go about interpreting the F ratios in the summary table.

All three F values are high, and the associated p values are very small; that is, all three are statistically significant. These results confirm the strong indications from the graph that:

- being taught the mnemonic strategy improves retention, *irrespective of time* (main effect of Strategy);

- memory deteriorates progressively over time, *irrespective of strategy* (main effect of Days); and

- the rate of deterioration of memory is faster for the group without the training ((Strategy × Days) interaction).

These effects can be 'unpicked' further using Tukey's HSD test (see Figure 13.10) and the main effect of Days can be investigated through a **linear trend test** (see Figure 13.9, ANOVA summary table).

BEFORE READING ON . . .

Think about the (Strategy × Days) interaction. Is there another way of expressing the nature of this interaction? Jot down your thoughts.

. . . now read on

An alternative way of describing the interaction between strategy and time would be to say that the magnitude of the strategy effect differs depending on time elapsed – specifically, the effect of strategy is greater as the time elapsed

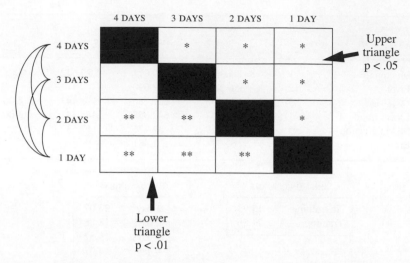

Figure 13.10 *Fading memories* – Tukey's HSD tests

increases. Remember, again, that this is simply another way of expressing the same idea and, while it may seem to be labouring the point in this case, there may be occasions when it is necessary to look at patterns of interaction from more than one perspective in order to understand them fully.

SETTLING MORE DIFFERENCES

A further useful set of follow-up tests goes by the name of **Simple Effects**. What this approach does is to look at the effects of each factor, not overall, but *separately* for each level of the other factor. Think of simple effects as a series of *mini ANOVAs*.

In our example, we can look at the effects of the experimental condition (*training* or *no training*) separately after 1 day, after 2 days, after 3 days, and after 4 days. Conversely, we can look at the effects of time elapsed for the control group and the experimental group separately. These two versions of simple effects reflect the above exercise of describing our interaction from two perspectives. The result is a bunch of F ratios, which are summarised in Figure 13.11.

Thus, the experimental treatment has a significant effect whether the time elapsed is 1 day, 2 days, 3 days or 4 days. However, note the increasing F ratios, reflecting the trend visible in the graph that the separation between the groups increases over time (this is what constitutes the interaction, in fact). Similarly, looking at the interaction the other way round, time elapsed is significant for both the control group and the experimental group separately.

Note that, when factors have only two levels, simple effects allow unambiguous interpretation. For factors with more than two levels, however, they may need to be used in conjunction with multiple comparisons, such as Tukey's HSD

SIMPLE EFFECT	F	df	p
Mnemonic at 1 Day	6.801	1,17	.018
Mnemonic at 2 Days	193.143	1,17	.000
Mnemonic at 3 Days	257.143	1,17	.000
Mnenomic at 4 Days	468.643	1,17	.000
Days at No training	210.714	3,36	.000
Days at Training	45.048	3,36	.000

Figure 13.11 *Fading memories* – simple effects

test, since the various levels of the factor(s) may need to be unpicked in order to reveal the source of an interaction.

BEFORE READING ON . . .

Spend some time thinking about this last point. Make sure you understand when it might be necessary to use multiple comparisons in conjunction with simple effects.

. . . now read on

FAME AND RECOGNITION

Figure 13.12 again presents a graph for the data about recognition of photographs by male and female students (between factor) for three categories of photo (within

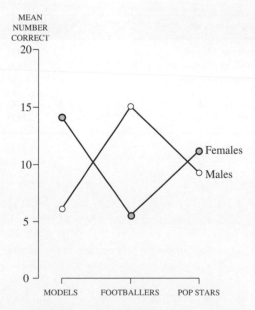

Figure 13.12 *Fame and recognition* – identification scores by gender and type of photograph

factor). Looking at the ANOVA summary table (Figure 13.13), we see no main effects, but a huge F ratio for the interaction. This is in line with what the graph, and the patterns of means, suggest strongly.

SOURCE OF VARIATION	df	SUM OF SQUARES	MEAN SQUARE	F	p
Gender	1	.167	.167	.009	.9255
Error	16	295.704	18.481		
Photo category	2	.481	.241	.100	.9048
GP interaction	2	714.778	357.389	149.027	.0000
Error	32	76.741	2.398		

GENDER MEANS	
Male	10.19
Female	10.30

PHOTO CATEGORY MEANS	
Models	10.11
Footballers	10.33
Pop stars	10.28

Figure 13.13 ANOVA summary table for *Fame and recognition* example

The impressions are further confirmed by carrying out tests for simple effects, with the results as shown in Figure 13.14. Note the statistically significant differences between males and females for both models and footballers (note too that the differences are in opposite directions) but a non-significant difference for pop stars. Note also that the differences between categories – which were non-significant for the main effect – are statistically significant when males and females are looked at separately.

SIMPLE EFFECT	F	df	p
Gender at Models	37.117	1,25	.000
Gender at Footballers	52.955	1,25	.000
Gender at Pop stars	2.069	1,25	.163
Category at Male	78.039	2,32	.000
Category at Female	71.089	2,32	.000

Figure 13.14 *Fame and recognition* – simple effects

Student: I can see I shall have to be careful in interpreting ANOVA summary tables. When I first looked at this one, I thought there were no effects of either Gender or Category, and that was more or less end of story.

Statistician: It's certainly true that, in a formal sense, the main effects of Gender and Category are not even approaching significance, but the highly significant interaction hides a multitude! In fact, it is completely obscuring strong effects of both Gender and Category.

Student: So any time I see a significant interaction, an alarm bell should ring?

Statistician: Absolutely. If you have a significant interaction you must look at the data in more detail.

Student: Precisely how should I go about it?

Statistician: As our example illustrates very well, the obvious first step is to draw a graph. Spend some time looking at it in order to get a sense of the nature of the interaction – maybe even plot the two versions of the graph. Then choose appropriate follow-up tests formally to confirm or disconfirm your conclusions about the true nature of your results.

Student: So, if I want to know if some means differ significantly from others, I would choose multiple comparisons or simple effects?

Statistician: Or sometimes both, and if you were interested in, say, a linear trend, you would test for that.

Student: Life would be much simpler if interactions were not significant.

Statistician: Indeed, but much less interesting as well!

HOT AND BOTHERED

Figure 13.15 presents the graph for the example about the effects of noise level (a within factor, remember) and temperature (also a within factor) on typing performance. The summary table this time (Figure 13.16) has three error terms, because the ANOVA design is **two-factor within** (again, it is beyond our aims of this book to explain why).

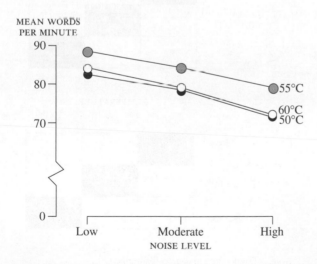

Figure 13.15 *Hot and bothered* – typing speed (wpm) by noise and temperature

In this example, consistent with the patterns evident in the graph, both main effects are statistically significant, but the interaction between the factors does not produce a statistically significant effect. This allows for a much more straightforward interpretation of the main effects, since the absence of interaction means that the effect of noise level is the same for all three levels of temperature. Also the effect of temperature is the same for all noise levels.

SOURCE OF VARIATION	df	SUM OF SQUARES	MEAN SQUARE	F	p
Subjects	7	1246.667	178.095		
Noise level	2	1569.778	784.889	161.595	.0000
Error	14	68.000	4.857		
Temperature	2	444.111	222.056	30.780	.0000
Error	14	101.000	7.214		
NT interaction	4	3.556	.889	.330	.8552
Error	28	75.333	2.690		

NOISE LEVEL MEANS

Low	85.00
Moderate	80.67
High	73.67

TEMPERATURE MEANS

50°C	77.58
55°C	83.25
60°C	78.50

Figure 13.16 ANOVA summary table for *Hot and bothered* example

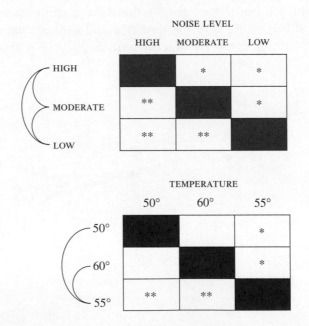

Note: Temperature in degrees Fahrenheit

Figure 13.17 Hot and bothered – Tukey's HSD tests

The results of Tukey HSD tests are as shown in Figure 13.17. Here, the means for each main effect have been compared separately; that is, averaging across the levels of the other factor. We could have performed Tukey tests on all nine means shown in the graph (known as the **interaction means**), but this would have produced a 9 × 9 table of comparisons. We can avoid having to produce such an unwieldy analysis because the interaction was not significant in this case. Had there been a significant interaction, we would have needed to compare the interaction means.

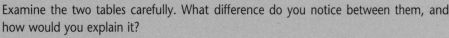

BEFORE READING ON . . .

Examine the two tables carefully. What difference do you notice between them, and how would you explain it?

As an exercise, plot and interpret the graph 'the other way around'; that is, with temperature along the horizontal axis and a separate line for each level of noise. Does this help you explain the difference between the two Tukey tables?

. . . now read on

PICTURES IN THE MIND

In the final example (Figure 13.18), the graph shows a consistently longer decision time for reversed figures, and a clear relationship between the angle of rotation and the decision time. (Again, it's a two-*factor within design*).

The ANOVA table is shown in Figure 13.19. It confirms that both the main effects are statistically significant, but not the interaction. Again, you will see that, because it is a two-factor within design, each systematic source of variation has

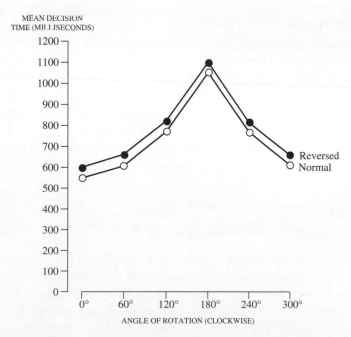

Figure 13.18 *Pictures in the mind* – response time (msec.) by angle and type

SOURCE OF VARIATION	df	SUM OF SQUARES	MEAN SQUARE	F	p
Subjects	5	31808.944	6361.789		
Type	1	43610.870	43610.870	5391.454	.0000
Error	5	40.444	8.089		
Angle	5	2005779.123	401155.825	4578.591	.0000
Error	25	2190.389	87.616		
TA interaction	5	16.778	3.356	.542	.7429
Error	25	154.889	6.196		

TYPE	MEANS
Normal	727.36
Reversed	776.58

ANGLE	MEANS
0°	576.08
60°	634.58
120°	793.50
180°	1077.42
240°	792.83
300°	637.42

Figure 13.19 ANOVA summary table for *Pictures in the mind* example

its own separate error term. This is different from the two-factor mixed design, which in turn is different from the two-factor between design. Remember that, irrespective of the number of error terms, the principles governing the interpretation of F ratios associated with the systematic sources of variation are identical in all cases.

As in the previous example, the absence of an interaction permits a straightforward interpretation of the main effects. Since there is a significant main effect of Type (and no interaction), we can conclude that the effect of Type is pretty much the same for all levels of Angle. Similarly, we can conclude that the effect of Angle is the same for both levels of Type.

Since there are only two levels of Type, follow-up analysis is redundant. The nature of differences between the different angles can be investigated using Tukey's HSD test. Additionally, while a trend test across all six levels of Angle would not produce evidence of a linear trend, separate trend tests for 0–180 and 180–300 would be likely to reveal highly significant linear trends.

CHAPTER REVIEW

This chapter has gone through the same examples as in the previous chapter, but this time looking at the ANOVA results for statistical significance or otherwise, and introducing various follow-up methods that help to tease out the details of the salient patterns in the data. Careful study of these examples will pay dividends – noting the relationships between the raw data and various derived means, graphical representations, and the results from the ANOVA tables and follow-up tests. Everything contributes to the art of interpreting the evidence.

Relating: Multiple variables

... the topic of regression analysis is extended beyond the simple case introduced in Chapter 8. Paralleling the extension of ANOVA from one to more than one independent variables, multiple regression analysis (MRA) allows the relationship between several independent variables and a dependent variable to be investigated. Following an introduction to the concept of a *regression model*, a variety of examples are presented, illustrating the flexibility of the technique. Contrasts between ANOVA and MRA are discussed briefly.

INTRODUCING MULTIPLE REGRESSION ANALYSIS

In Chapter 8, we introduced the idea of fitting a regression line to a scatterplot showing the relationship between two variables. When these two variables are correlated and related in a more-or-less linear fashion (as a scatterplot will show), the fitted line summarises the relationship between them – the closer the correlation to ±1, the more exact the relationship, the closer to 0, the less linear. Now we shall show how this form of analysis can be extended to examine the relationship among more than two variables – analogously to the extension within ANOVA to more than one factor.

The initial example for this purpose concerns a study of what characteristics of students may affect their performance on a practical statistics test in which they are asked to use a statistical package to carry out analysis of provided data and to interpret the results. The specific aspects to be considered are measured IQ, attitudes to computers, and amount of time spent practising with the software. Figure 14.1 presents the data (note that these are not authentic data, but have been constructed to be at least plausible, and to provide a suitable example for our purposes).

To begin with, we can consider the variables *IQ*, Attitudes to Computers (*Attitudes*, for short), and Amount of Practice (*Practice*, for short) separately in relation

| PREDICTOR VARIABLES | | | CRITERION VARIABLE |
IQ	ATTITUDE TO COMPUTERS	HOURS OF PRACTICE	MARK
121	49	10	61
106	43	14	58
140	41	34	67
111	60	22	41
121	41	9	44
124	56	6	52
104	52	13	46
131	56	17	75
130	61	27	72
138	47	8	25
137	53	12	66
128	45	18	54
127	64	31	85
117	57	21	60
129	56	23	62
113	44	14	30
143	46	11	20
138	54	24	54

.582

.490

.054

Correlations with criterion variable

Figure 14.1 IQ, *Attitudes*, *Practice* and test performance (*Mark*)

to performance on the test (*Mark*), in terms of the product-moment correlation coefficients, shown at the bottom of Figure 14.1. For $N = 18$, the critical value for r is .468, so the correlations of *Attitudes* with *Mark*, and *Practice* with *Mark* are both statistically significant at the .05 level. The correlation between *IQ* and *Mark* is low, and not statistically significant.

The next step is to examine how *IQ*, *Attitudes* and *Practice* relate to *Mark*, *collectively* rather than separately. Traditionally, in such a case, *IQ*, *Attitudes*, and *Practice* are called **predictor variables**, and *Mark* is called the **criterion variable**. Simple Regression Analysis, described in Chapter 8, deals with the relationship between one predictor variable and a criterion variable. As an extension, Multiple Regression Analysis is concerned with the relationship between a set of predictor variables amalgamated in a way we shall describe below, and a criterion variable.

To work through this extension, we'll start with the combination of *Attitudes* and *Practice*. The standard method used is to form a combination of the general form:

$$Y' = a + b_1X_1 + b_2X_2$$

where a, b_1 and b_2, are specific numbers, and X_1 and X_2 are two predictor variables. Before we explain how the numbers a, b_1 and b_2 are determined, consider how this equation resembles the simpler case of the straight-line equation from Chapter 8:

$$Y' = a + bX$$

where a is the intercept and b the slope. Note that when this notation was introduced, it wasn't necessary to number either the slope, b, or the predictor variable, X, since there was only one of each. You should be able to see that the more complex formula is just a generalisation of the simpler one. For the more complex formula:

$$Y' = a + b_1X_1 + b_2X_2$$

the meaning of the intercept, a, generalises in the sense that it is the value of Y' when X_1 and X_2 are both zero. The slopes, b_1 and b_2, are the increases in Y' for every unit increase in X_1 and X_2, respectively.

The mathematics, as you might expect, is more complicated than it is for the case of simple regression. However, the same basic principle applies. Think of Y' as a new variable constructed by amalgamating X_1 and X_2 according to the general formula – with the numbers a, b_1 and b_2 open to us to choose according to whatever criterion we apply. A standard criterion that is adopted is to choose those precise values of a, b_1 and b_2 that will make Y' as good an approximation to Y as possible in the sense that $\Sigma(Y' - Y)^2$ is as small as possible. This method is called the method of **least squares**, since it minimises the sum of the squared differences between the actual values of the criterion variable and the values predicted by the formula. The least squares criterion is analogous to the criterion used in the simple case with a single predictor (see page 141).

Once this criterion is adopted, it can be shown – by mathematics that is not particularly complex – that the values of a, b_1 and b_2 are determined, and these values can be calculated. In practice, we do not expect you to be doing multiple regression without computer software, so we simply state that the equation that results for the example is:

$$Y' = -3.334 + .778X_1 + .995X_2$$

where X_1 is *Attitudes*, and X_2 is *Practice*.

Figure 14.2 lays out in some detail how this works. X_1 and X_2 are shown as columns, each column consisting of the eighteen values for the respective pre-

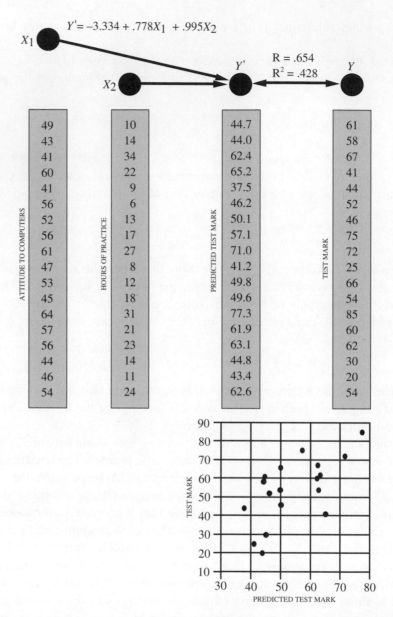

Figure 14.2 Predicting *Mark* from *Attitudes* and *Practice* – regression model and multiple correlation (*R*) between 'predicted *Mark*' and *Mark*

dictor variable. On the right is the criterion variable *Y*, similarly represented as a column containing the values for that variable, *Mark*. The data are aligned, participant by participant; that is, the data in any given row are for the same person. *Y'* is formed by amalgamating X_1 and X_2 according to the formula. Specifically, this works by applying the formula to each row of data in turn. For example, the first value of X_1 is 49, and the corresponding value of X_2 is 10. Putting those values into the formula:

$$Y' = -3.334 + (.778 \times 49) + (.995 \times 10)$$

gives a corresponding value of 44.7 (to 1 decimal place) for Y' for the first participant listed. The rest of the data for the column Y' are calculated in the same way.

BEFORE READING ON . . .

Check for yourself several more values of Y', using the formula.

. . . now read on

To see how closely Y' relates to Y, we can use a scatterplot, as shown in the figure, and calculate the correlation between them. Here we see that there is a moderately strong positive correlation between Y' and Y. Because Y' is formed from multiple predictors (in this case, two), this correlation is called a **multiple correlation**, and **R** is used as notation for it. Here R = .654, and its square R^2 = .428 – the significance of considering R^2, and not simply R, will appear shortly. (Note that R^2 is less than R, which will always be the case for R lying between 0 and 1 – make sure that you understand why this is necessarily the case).

We shall use the term **regression model** to refer to a regression equation with one or more predictors, and the associated multiple correlation between Y' and Y, and represent it as in Figure 14.3. We can test for statistical significance of such a model using a statistic defined in general as follows:

$$F = \frac{R^2/m}{(1 - R^2)/(N - m - 1)}$$

where m is the number of predictors, and N is the number of cases. In our example, replacing the general components of the formula R^2, m, N with their particular values .428, 2, 18, respectively, this works out as follows:

$$F = \frac{.428/2}{(1 - .428)/(18 - 2 - 1)} = 5.612$$

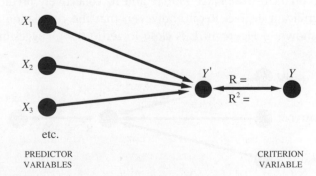

etc.

PREDICTOR
VARIABLES

CRITERION
VARIABLE

Figure 14.3 Regression model

This F statistic is, in fact, the statistic as used in ANOVA. As with ANOVA, the F statistic here has two associated degrees of freedom, which are given by the general formula $(m, N - m - 1)$, becoming $(2,15)$ for the example. The obtained value of F, 5.612, with these degrees of freedom, is statistically significant.

What does statistical significance mean here? As usual, it refers to the probability of getting a value of the statistic as extreme as that actually obtained from the data, if the null hypothesis is true. Here the null hypothesis, roughly speaking, is that the predictors, collectively, are not related to the criterion. If the null hypothesis is true, the probability of the F ratio (taking into account the degrees of freedom) exceeding 3.68 is .05 (3.68 being the critical value for 2, 15 degrees of freedom). If that critical value is exceeded (which happens in this case) then the result is statistically significant at the .05 level.

In practice, as is the usual story, the software you use is likely to give an exact probability (p). In this case, p = .015, which means that, if the null hypothesis is true, the probability of a value of F as extreme as 5.612 is .015 (and since this is less than .05, the result is statistically significant at the .05 level).

Now let's consider what happens if *IQ* is also included as a predictor. For three predictors, as you might expect, the general form of the regression equation is:

$$Y' = a + b_1X_1 + b_2X_2 + b_3X_3$$

with a, b_1, b_2, b_3 determined so as to minimise $\Sigma(Y' - Y)^2$ in a way that parallels the cases with one or two predictors.

For this example, with *Attitudes*, *Practice* and *IQ* as predictors of *Mark*, the relationship between the variables is shown by the model in Figure 14.4.

BEFORE READING ON . . .

Work out the F ratio, and associated degrees of freedom, for this model.

. . . now read on

You should get F = 3.497, with (3, 14) degrees of freedom. This is statistically significant at the .05 level (the exact p value being .0442).

So the three predictors, *Attitudes*, *Practice* and *IQ* collectively predict *Mark* to a statistically significant degree. Recall, however, that the correlation between *IQ* and *Mark*, as shown in Figure 14.1, is close to zero (.054), suggesting that *IQ* is

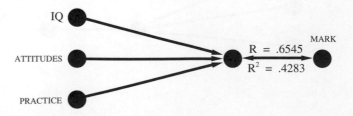

IQ

MARK

R = .6545

ATTITUDES

R^2 = .4283

PRACTICE

Figure 14.4 Regression model for predicting *Mark* from *Attitudes*, *Practice* and IQ

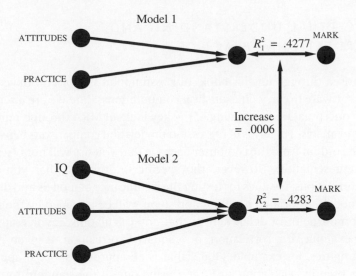

Figure 14.5 Predicting *Mark* – assessing the predictive power of IQ by comparing 2- and 3-predictor models

not an important determinant of *Mark*. The low value of this correlation suggests that *IQ* is not 'pulling its weight' in terms of the 3-predictor model, and that it is essentially *Attitudes* and *Practice* that are providing the *predictive power*. We can analyse this apparent pattern by comparing the 3-predictor model with the previous 2-predictor model.

Figure 14.5 shows us that the addition of *IQ* as a third predictor increases R^2 by only a very small amount. We can test for the statistical significance of this increase by using the formula:

$$F = \frac{(R_2^2 - R_1^2)/k}{(1 - R_2^2)/(N - (m + k) - 1)}$$

where *m* is the number of predictors in the first model and *k* is the number of extra predictors in the more inclusive model.

BEFORE READING ON . . .

Work out the F ratio, and associated degrees of freedom, for the comparison of the two models, by substituting the particular values in the general formula.

. . . now read on

You should get F = .0164, with (1,14) df, which is nowhere close to being statistically significant. The appropriate interpretation is that *IQ* does not add significantly to the predictive power already produced by *Attitudes* and *Practice*.

CONCEPTUAL UNDERSTANDING AND COMPUTATIONAL PRACTICE

As emphasised throughout this book, our assumption is that you have access to computer software to carry out statistical computations. Here we are attempting to provide a conceptual understanding of the key ideas of MRA through representing the results of analyses in terms of regression models and comparisons between such models. The output from the computer package that you use will not resemble this form of representation. However, the specific information that you need on multiple correlations, F values for testing the significance of models and differences between models, associated p values, and so on, will be provided by the software.

An important point of detail here is that any calculations involve approximations. For example, if a correlation, or a squared correlation, is given even to 4 significant figures, for example, .3062, that is an approximation. If approximate figures are used in calculating an F ratio using one of the standard formulas (as done throughout this chapter) the result will be slightly inaccurate (technically known as rounding error). Thus, if you re-analyse the data for some examples with a computer package – which works to a much more exact approximation – the values of F that it produces will differ slightly from those given here (as well as being more accurate).

AN ANALOGY

At this point, we introduce an analogy that we hope may give you some intuitive feeling for how a regression equation works. Imagine eleven people turning out their pockets to see how much cash they have, in terms of £1 coins, fifty-pence (50p) pieces, twenty-pence (20p) pieces, and smaller change. The data are shown in Figure 14.6.

NUMBER OF £1 COINS	NUMBER OF 50P	NUMBER OF 20P	CHANGE (IN PENCE)	TOTAL (IN PENCE)
3	3	2	15	505
12	8	3	25	1685
4	1	4	21	551
6	4	2	26	866
8	7	3	7	1217
8	2	1	18	938
5	10	6	14	1134
6	3	4	7	837
7	1	2	27	817
2	5	3	39	549
0	3	3	4	214

Figure 14.6 Breakdown of cash in pocket – low many £1 coins, 50p pieces, 20p pieces and smaller coins (10p or less)?

You should be able to reason that the number of £1 coins is a major determinant of the total amount of money, so the correlation between number of pounds and total amount should be high. The number of 50p pieces is less important in determining the total, but still has some bearing on it, so the correlation of that with total amount should be less. After that, the correlations should become small. The actual correlations are as shown in Figure 14.7.

	CORRELATION WITH TOTAL AMOUNT
NUMBER OF £1 COINS	.9207
NUMBER OF 50P	.6479
NUMBER OF 20P	.1342
CHANGE	.0799

Figure 14.7 Correlations between numbers of each coin and total cash in pocket

Now consider a sequence of regression models in which total amount of money is treated as the criterion variable and the other variables are added sequentially in as predictors (see Figure 14.8). The number of pounds already correlates highly with total amount of money. Adding in number of 50p pieces as a second predictor increases the value of R^2 to .9974, and adding the number of 20p pieces as a third predictor increases R^2 further to .9994 (getting very close to 1). For practice in using the formula, you might like to see if these increases are statistically significant.

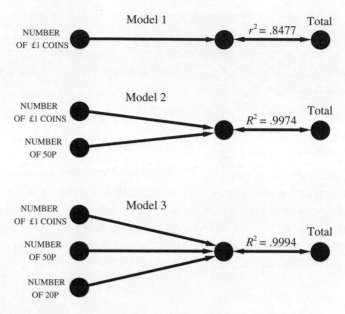

Figure 14.8 Predicting total cash from coinage – three regression models

The total amount of money (in pence) is given *exactly* by the formula:

total = (100 × number of £1 coins)
    + (50 × number of 50p pieces)
    + (20 × number of 20p pieces)
    + (1 × amount of small change),

so in this case, Y' and Y would be identical, there would be a perfect multiple correlation and R^2 would be 1.

If you think carefully about the different components in this analogy and how they are related logically, it should help to give you a feel for what is going on in MRA.

VARIATIONS ON THE MULTIPLE REGRESSION ANALYSIS THEME

A wide variety of useful forms of analysis can be carried out using the basic repertoire we have introduced in terms of regression models and significance tests for either (a) a single regression model; or (b) the comparison between two regression models, one of which contains a subset of the predictor variables in the other. In this section, we illustrate this variety with a number of examples.

CATEGORY VARIABLES AS PREDICTORS

In order to use a category (or *nominal*) variable (see page 20) as a predictor variable in MRA, special steps need to be taken.

Here are some fictitious data for sense of humour, measured on a scale from 0 to 100 (you might like to think about how sense of humour could be measured in practice) for twenty individuals belonging to four different nationalities, which, to avoid possible offence, we have labelled, but not identified (see Figure 14.9).

| | NATIONALITY | | | |
	A	B	C	D
	82	42	52	62
	61	66	53	59
	57	61	39	72
	63	50	67	75
	64		54	69
			48	
Means	65.4	54.8	52.2	67.4

Figure 14.9 Sense of humour by nationality

What must NOT be done is to code nationalities A, B, C, D as 1, 2, 3, 4 and treat this as a single predictor variable.

BEFORE READING ON . . .

Think about why doing the above would be silly.

. . . now read on

Coding nationality within a single predictor variable as 1, 2, 3, 4 would imply that the four nationalities are ordered and, more specifically, that the differences between A and B, B and C, C and D are all equal. No such ordered relationship exists. The appropriate way to treat nationality, or any other category variable, as a predictor for MRA is to recode the data by introducing so-called **dummy variables**. Figure 14.10 shows how this works for our example.

There are three dummy variables. The first takes the value 1 if that individual's nationality is A, and the value 0 otherwise. The second and third relate in a similar way to nationalities B and C, respectively. You might be expecting a fourth dummy variable for nationality D, but in fact it is not necessary, because any individual coded as 0, 0, 0 for the three dummy variables must of necessity be of

DUMMY 1	DUMMY 2	DUMMY 3	HUMOUR SCORE
1	0	0	82
1	0	0	61
1	0	0	57
1	0	0	63
1	0	0	64
0	1	0	42
0	1	0	66
0	1	0	61
0	1	0	50
0	0	1	52
0	0	1	53
0	0	1	39
0	0	1	67
0	0	1	54
0	0	1	48
0	0	0	62
0	0	0	59
0	0	0	72
0	0	0	75
0	0	0	69

Figure 14.10 Recoding nationality – the use of dummy variables

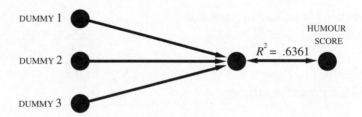

Figure 14.11 Predicting sense of humour from nationality through dummy variables

nationality D, by elimination. In general, *if a category variable has k categories, it is coded by k – 1 dummy variables.*

Having recoded the data in this way, the regression analysis proceeds as normal, with the dummy variables being treated as a set of predictors. (Even though these variables are dichotomous, coded as 0 as 1 for each individual, the standard formula for working out the regression equation, multiple correlation, F ratio for testing for significance, and so on, can be applied.) The resulting model is shown in Figure 14.11.

The F ratio to test for significance of the model is 3.625 with (3,16) df and this is significant at the .05 level (the exact p value is .0361). The appropriate interpretation is that we can reject the null hypothesis that the populations from the four nationalities do not differ in terms of sense of humour as measured. Note that this is a general statement, and does not pinpoint where differences exist between the nationalities. Eyeballing the means, it looks as if nationalities A and D have better senses of humour that nationalities B and C. In order to check this pattern of differences more precisely, some follow-up procedures would be needed (as is the case when a significant effect is found in ANOVA) but we're not going to cover that.

In any case where the variable is dichotomous – that is, can only take two values (for example, gender), the variable can be coded simply as a single predictor using 0 and 1 for the two categories (note that this is a special case of k categories requiring $k - 1$ dummy variables; when $k = 2$, $k - 1 = 1$).

The same data could have been analysed using ANOVA. If that is done, in fact, you finish up with the same value of F (and the same degrees of freedom), exemplifying the close link between the two statistical techniques. The example is intended to show how coding of dummy variables works in general; for example, for situations in which category variables are mixed with other sorts of variables in a regression analysis with several predictors, as will be illustrated in the next example.

SELECTING FROM MULTIPLE PREDICTORS

Next we look at a rather more complex example, using real data for 172 psychology students. A small part of the data is shown in Figure 14.12.

The question to be addressed by analysing these data is what variables predict students' attitudes towards computers (abbreviated to *Attitude*). The variables to be considered are Faculty (Arts, Science or Economics), Gender, IQ, External Locus of Control (a measure of the degree to which individuals consider that their

PREDICTOR VARIABLES					CRITERION VARIABLE
FACULTY	GENDER	IQ	EXTERNAL LoC	COMPUTER USE	ATTITUDE TO COMPUTERS
Science	Female	104	10	Yes	55
Economics	Female	107	10	Yes	58
Arts	Male	97	17	No	41
Economics	Female	97	17	No	43
Arts	Female	87	16	No	52
Science	Female	94	13	Yes	56
Arts	Male	93	16	Yes	61
Arts	Female	104	14	No	45
.	.	.	.	.	.
.	.	.	.	.	.
.	.	.	.	.	.
.	.	.	.	.	.

Figure 14.12 Faculty, Gender, IQ, External LoC, Computer use, and Attitude (to computers) – real data

behaviour is controlled by external events rather than under their own control – commonly abbreviated to External LoC), and Computer use (which, in this case, is simply the answer to the question: 'Have you done a computer course before?'). The first step is to recode Gender and Computer Use as 0s and 1s, and Faculty as 2 dummy variables, Fac1 and Fac2, with the result shown in Figure 14.13. When all variables are included as predictors, the model looks like that in Figure 14.14.

	PREDICTOR VARIABLES					CRITERION VARIABLE
FACULTY 1	FACULTY 2	GENDER	IQ	EXTERNAL LoC	COMPUTER USE	ATTITUDE TO COMPUTERS
0	1	1	104	10	1	55
0	0	1	107	10	1	58
1	0	0	97	17	0	41
0	0	1	97	17	0	43
1	0	1	87	16	0	52
0	1	1	94	13	1	56
1	0	0	93	16	1	61
1	0	1	104	14	0	45
•	•	•	•	•	•	•
•	•	•	•	•	•	•
•	•	•	•	•	•	•
•	•	•	•	•	•	•

Figure 14.13 Recoding Gender, Computer use and Faculty

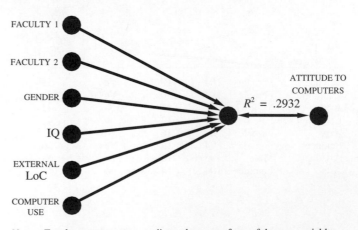

Note: Faculty counts as two predictors because of use of dummy variables

Figure 14.14 6-predictor regression model – predicting computer attitudes from Faculty, Gender, IQ, External LoC and Computer use

	CORRELATION WITH ATTITUDE TO COMPUTERS	SQUARED CORRELATION
FACULTY 1 + FACULTY 2	.0961	.0092
GENDER	.0706	.0050
IQ	.0533	.0028
EXTERNAL LoC	−.3136	.0983
COMPUTER USE	.4572	.2090

Figure 14.15 Separate correlations between attitude and the five variables

Separate correlations between each predictor variable and Attitude are as shown in Figure 14.15. For Gender, IQ, External LoC and Computer use, these are simple (bivariate) correlations. The correlation for Faculty consists of a multiple correlation produced by combining the two dummy variables.

So it looks as if External LoC and Computer use are the important predictors. (Note that the correlation between External LoC and Attitude is negative, indicating that, in general, a higher degree of External LoC goes with a lower attitude towards computers, and vice versa.) The dominance of the major predictors may be confirmed by comparing the model that contains just those two predictors with the original model containing the full set of predictors (Figure 14.16).

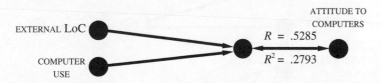

Figure 14.16 Predicting computer attitude using just External LoC and Computer use

The two predictors in this model give a value for R^2 of .2793, which is only marginally less than the value of .2932 given by the full set of predictors (see Figure 14.14). Note that the coefficient for X_1 (External LoC) in the regression equation is negative, reflecting the inverse relationship between this predictor and the criterion variable.

We may use this example to explain further how it is possible to test for **interaction** within MRA. By way of example, we shall show how to test for an interaction between External LoC and Computer use. What would an interaction mean in this case? It can be expressed in various ways, but perhaps the clearest would be to say that there would be an interaction if the relationship between External LoC and Attitude differed depending on whether or not the individual had previous experience of computers. This reflects the general meaning of an interaction between two variables, discussed extensively in relation to ANOVA (Chapters 10 to 13), that the effects of one variable differ depending on the value of the other variable.

In practical terms, the procedure for testing for a statistically significant interaction between two predictor variables, X_1 and X_2, goes as follows. A new variable is created by multiplying the value of X_1 by the value of X_2 for each individual. Then a comparison of models is carried out using the usual formula, the first model having X_1 and X_2 as predictors, and the second X_1, X_2 and X_1X_2. In the case of the example, the resulting models are as seen in Figure 14.17. You will see that adding X_1X_2 as an extra predictor increases the squared multiple correlation only slightly, and an F test will confirm that this small increase is far from statistically significant. We conclude therefore that there is no evidence in these data of an interaction between External LoC and Computer use.

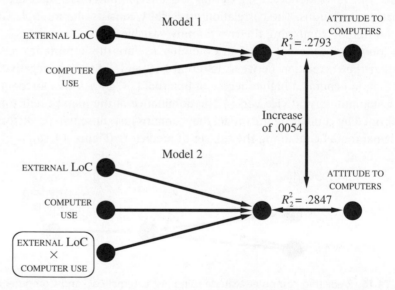

Figure 14.17 Investigating a possible interaction between External LoC and Computer use

THE COMPLICATION OF CORRELATED PREDICTORS: BURT DATA

To illustrate another key point about MRA, we return to the data from Burt's study (Figure 14.18) already analysed quite extensively in Chapter 8.

Given the generally high correlations between Poverty, Poor Relief and Overcrowding, separately, and Juvenile Delinquency – r = .66, .42 (ignoring the

BOROUGH	JUVENILE DELINQUENCY (PER 10,000)	POVERTY (BOOTH'S MEASURE)	POOR RELIEF (PER 1000)	PERCENTAGE OVERCROWDING
Finsbury	42	37	22	34
Holborn	36	49	16	20
Shoreditch	28	42	51	32
Bermondsey	23	44	46	23
St. Pancras	21	30	20	22
Southwark	18	49	32	24
Stepney	17	38	20	29
Battersea	16	38	43	12
Deptford	16	40	40	13
St. Marylebone	15	27	8	18
Westminster	15	35	5	10
Paddington	14	22	15	15
Bethnal Green	14	45	25	28
Islington	14	31	26	19
Hammersmith	13	34	17	14
Lambeth	12	26	21	13
Poplar	12	36	83	21
Kensington	12	25	10	17
Chelsea	12	25	13	14
Greenwich	11	37	16	14
Camberwell	10	29	34	13
Fulham	9	25	14	13
Woolwich	9	25	27	8
Hackney	8	24	18	12
Lewisham	7	18	23	5
City of London	5	32	4	7
Wandsworth	4	27	8	7
Hampstead	2	14	3	7
Stoke Newington	0	19	8	8

Figure 14.18 Burt's data on 'juvenile delinquency', poverty, poor relief and overcrowding

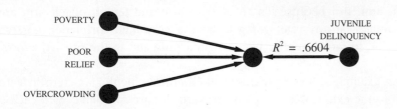

Figure 14.19 Regression model for predicting 'juvenile' delinquency' from poverty, poor relief and overcrowding

outlier) and .77, respectively (see Figure 8.18, on page 138) – and, given that it is plausible to consider the measures of poor social conditions as causally contributing to the level of Juvenile Delinquency, it would seem sensible to combine those three variables as predictors in an MRA, with Juvenile Delinquency as the criterion variable. Doing so produces the model in Figure 14.19.

So, the trio of predictors collectively predict Juvenile Delinquency to a considerable degree, with $R^2 = .660$ (which is statistically significant). But what if we want to tease the predictors apart and evaluate the importance of the contribu-

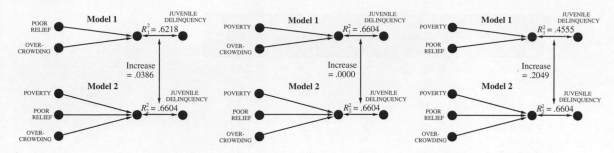

Figure 14.20 Teasing apart individual predictons from multiple regression (Burt data)

tion of each one independently? The contribution of any one predictor that can be *uniquely* attributed to that predictor can be found by comparing two models – one that contains all the predictors, and another that contains all of them except the one under consideration. Figure 14.20 shows the result for the Burt data.

The result is not straightforward to interpret. Overcrowding is the only one of the three that *adds* significantly to the amount of predictive power produced by the other two. Does this mean that it is the only one that predicts Juvenile Delinquency? This would be an odd conclusion to reach, since the other two also have high correlations, when correlated separately with Juvenile Delinquency.

The explanation lies in the fact that in this example the criterion variables are all highly correlated, not just with the criterion variable, but with each other (again, see Figure 8.18, on page 138). To get a feel for the implications of this pattern, consider the following glaringly obvious example. Suppose that, for a sample of individuals, you were using measurements of body parts to predict height. Length of left arm would be a very good predictor. So would length of right arm. But because length of right arm and length of left arm are (for most samples, at any rate) going to have a very high correlation – extremely close to +1, in fact – neither would significantly add to the predictive power of the other.

So this example shows dramatically another prominent characteristic feature of MRA – to the extent that the predictor variables are correlated with each other, their separate effects are difficult to tease apart. In this respect, MRA stands in marked contrast to ANOVA. For an ANOVA with equal numbers in each cell of the design, the analysis neatly parcels the variance into separate chunks – so much for each main effect, so much for each interaction, and so much unexplained (error variance).

ONE MORE EXAMPLE: ANALYSIS OF COVARIANCE

MRA is very flexible and has many specific useful applications, and one in particular is illustrated in this last example. The data are made up to illustrate four different possible patterns of results, but the basic structure of the experimental design is one that occurs frequently in applied research.

Consider a situation where two methods of teaching arithmetic are being compared – we'll call them Method A and Method B. Because this sort of study is done in a school and not a laboratory, the children being taught would usually not be assigned randomly to the two conditions. Instead, two existing classes are likely to be used – we'll call them Class A (taught by Method A) and Class B (taught by Method B). Many different methodologies could be brought to bear to investigate in detail the relative efficacy of the two teaching methods, but for our purposes we consider a simple form of design incorporating a *pre-test* (the children's ability in arithmetic is measured before the teaching takes place) and a *post-test* (their ability is measured again after the teaching takes place).

BEFORE READING ON . . .

You could compare the two methods by doing a t-test to compare the scores of the two classes on the post-test. Would this be reasonable? If not, why not?

. . . now read on

The problem about simply comparing the post-test scores is that if there is a statistically significant difference showing, for example, that Class A performed better on the Post-test than Class B, it could be attributable to Method A being more effective, or it could be attributable to the children in Class A being better at arithmetic to begin with (or both). Conversely, failure to find a significant difference when Method A is 'really' better than Method B could be because the children in Class B were better at arithmetic to begin with.

BEFORE READING ON . . .

Think very carefully through the logic and the implications of the two scenarios just described.

. . . now read on

The point of carrying out a pre-test now becomes apparent. It can be used to adjust statistically for any initial differences between the classes in arithmetic ability. A simple way to do this would be to work out, for each child, the difference between pre-test and post-test scores, representing the improvement during the teaching. These improvement scores could then be compared for the two classes.

	DATA SET 1		DATA SET 2		DATA SET 3		DATA SET 4	
	PRE-	POST-	PRE-	POST-	PRE-	POST-	PRE-	POST-
CLASS A	22	19	22	27	14	19	30	27
	23	30	23	38	15	30	31	38
	33	35	33	43	25	35	41	43
	29	25	29	33	21	25	37	33
	19	24	19	32	11	24	27	32
	12	15	12	23	4	15	20	23
	13	22	13	30	5	22	21	30
	20	31	28	39	20	31	36	39
CLASS B	16	18	16	18	16	18	16	18
	18	27	18	27	18	27	18	27
	34	32	34	32	34	32	34	32
	30	37	30	37	30	37	30	37
	26	21	26	21	26	21	26	21
	19	23	19	23	19	23	19	23
	10	17	10	17	10	17	10	17
	25	28	25	28	25	28	25	28

Figure 14.21 Illustrating the use of pre-test as a covariate – four contrasting data sets

A more sophisticated method of taking the pre-test scores into consideration is called **Analysis of Covariance**. A **covariate**, in general, is some variable that, for one reason or another, cannot be controlled for in carrying out the experiment (for example, by random assignment of participants to conditions) but which can be measured and so taken into account in the statistical analysis. *Prevention is better than cure, so to speak, but if prevention isn't possible, then cure is advisable.*

To make important points about Analysis of Covariance, four possible data sets are to be contrasted (see Figure 14.21). To work out what's going on in each case, it's helpful to have scatterplots for the four data sets, showing the relationship between pre-test and post-test scores for Class A and Class B (see Figure 14.22). Additionally, on the right-hand side in each case, a representation of the differences in post-test scores alone is provided.

BEFORE READING ON . . .

Look carefully at each of the plots and consider what the data in each case suggest about the relative efficacy of the two teaching methods.

. . . now read on

We now analyse each of the data sets in turn.

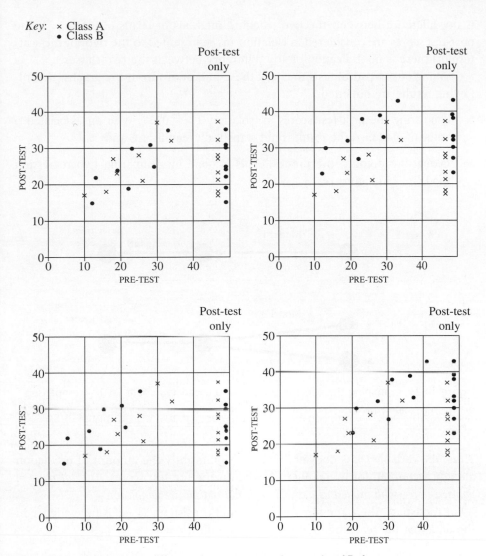

Note: Each graph also shows differences in post-test scores between A and B classes

Figure 14.22 Scatterplots of post-test against pre-test for the four data sets

Data set 1

The scatterplot shows that there is a clear correlation between pre-test scores and post-test scores, which is not surprising, if you think about it – students who are relatively good/poor to begin with are likely to remain relatively good/poor after instruction. Also, by taking into account the diagonal line through points with equal pre-test and post-test scores, it is clear that in most cases (all but three, to be precise) the post-test score is higher. Thus, these data indicate that the effects of the teaching in both classes have generally been positive. There is considerable overlap between the two sets of points within the scatterplot, suggesting that there is no difference between the two teaching methods in terms of efficacy. If the post-test scores are considered in isolation (as represented to the right of the scatterplot) there is no indication of any difference between the two classes.

Carrying out statistical tests to check these indications from the graphs, the following results are obtained:

- comparing the post-test scores in isolation: $t = -.0737$, with an associated p value of .9423, so the result is not statistically significant; and

- taking into account the pre-test. This is done by comparing two regression models, as in Figure 14.23.

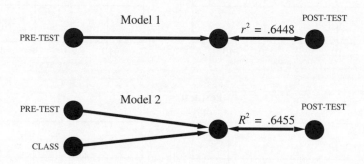

Figure 14.23 Examining the effect of pre-test as a covariate in data set 1 – comparison of two regression models

Thus, the variable Class does not increase significantly the amount of prediction already accounted for by taking into account the pre-test scores. *The difference in post-test scores, with pre-test as a covariate, is not statistically significant.*

For these data, then, the picture is clear and consistent. There is no evidence in the data that the teaching methods differ in efficacy.

Data set 2

The scatterplot again shows that there is a clear correlation between pre-test scores and post-test scores. Except for two cases, the post-test score is higher in each case. By contrast, there is now a strong visual suggestion of a difference between the two classes, with the points for Class A generally higher than those for Class B. A similar pattern is evident in the post-test scores considered in isolation.

Carrying out statistical tests to check these indications from the graphs, the following results are obtained:

- comparing the post-test scores: $t = 2.284$ with an associated p value of .0385, so the result is statistically significant at the .05 level; and

- taking into account the pre-test as covariate by comparing two regression models, as in Figure 14.24.

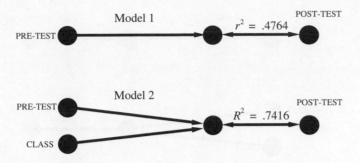

Figure 14.24 Examining the effect of pre-test as a covariate in data set 2 – comparison of two regression models

The variable Class significantly increases the amount of prediction already accounted for by taking into account the pre-test scores. In other words, *the difference in post-test scores, with pre-test as a covariate, is statistically significant.*

Again, the results from both tests point to the same conclusion – students in Class A did better on the post-test, and their performance was statistically significantly better even when pre-test marks were taken into account.

Data set 3

The scatterplot yet again shows that there is a clear correlation between pre-test scores and post-test scores for each class. With two exceptions, the post-test score is higher. As for the previous data set, there is a strong visual suggestion of a difference between the two classes, with the points for Class A generally higher than those for Class B. However, the same pattern is *not* evident in the post-test scores considered in isolation.

Carrying out statistical tests to check these indications from the graphs, the following results are obtained:

■ comparing the post-test scores: t = −.0737 with an associated p value of .9423, so the result is not statistically significant; and

■ taking into account the pre-test as covariate by comparing two regression models, as in Figure 14.25.

The variable Class significantly increases the amount of prediction already accounted for by taking into account the pre-test scores. In other words, *the difference in post-test scores, with pre-test as a covariate, is statistically significant.*

BEFORE READING ON . . .

Given that the t-test yields a result that is not statistically significant, and the Analysis of Covariance a result that is statistically significant, which should be followed? Why?

. . . *now read on*

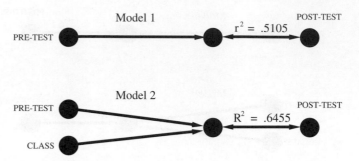

Figure 14.25 Examining the effect of pre-test as a covariate in data set 3 – comparison of two regression models

The Analysis of Covariance is the appropriate analysis in this case. The lack of a significant result for the t-test may be explained by examining the data in the scatterplot. It is true that the post-test scores for the two classes are similar overall, but the pre-test scores for Class A are, on average, considerably lower. Thus, the children in Class A have, in fact, shown greater improvement. This example is intended to show one way in which relying on the post-test scores alone would be misleading, and how the Analysis of Covariance, taking pre-test scores into account as well, avoids this problem.

Data set 4

As usual, the scatterplot shows a clear correlation between pre-test scores and post-test scores. Apart from four cases, the post-test score is higher. There is no hint in the scatterplot of a difference between the two classes. However, the same pattern is *not* evident in the post-test scores considered in isolation, where there appears to be a clear difference.

Carrying out statistical tests to check these indications from the graphs, the following results are obtained:

■ comparing the post-test scores: t = 2.284 with an associated p value of .0385, so the result is statistically significant; and

■ taking into account the pre-test as covariate by comparing two regression models, as in Figure 14.26.

The variable Class does not significantly increase the amount of prediction already accounted for by taking into account the pre-test scores. In other words, *the difference in post-test scores, with pre-test as a covariate, is not statistically significant.*

BEFORE READING ON . . .

Given that the t-test yields a result that is statistically significant, and the Analysis of Covariance a result that is not statistically significant, which should be followed? Why?

. . . now read on

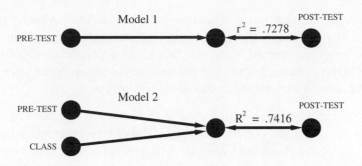

Figure 14.26 Examining the effect of pre-test as a covariate in data set 4 – comparison of two regression models

The Analysis of Covariance is again the appropriate analysis. The significant result for the t-test may be explained by examining the data in the scatterplot. It is true that the post-test scores for the two classes differ overall, but the pre-test scores for Class A are, on average, considerably higher. Thus, the children in Class A have, in fact, shown no greater improvement than those in Class B – they started higher, and they finished higher. This example is intended to show another way in which relying on the post-test scores would be misleading, and how the Analysis of Covariance, taking pre-test scores into account as well, avoids this problem.

THE RELATIVE STRENGTHS AND WEAKNESSES OF MRA AND ANOVA

The first example presented in this chapter gives us a convenient starting point to make some comments about the contrasting characteristics of MRA and ANOVA. In that example, we showed how to analyse the relationship between Attitudes, Practice and IQ as predictor variables, and Mark as the criterion variable, using MRA. These data could be analysed using ANOVA but before this could be done they would need to be converted into a form that fits the ANOVA mould. Consider IQ, for example. It can be used as a factor in ANOVA, but only if expressed in terms of a relatively small number of levels. For example, we could define High, Medium and Low IQ as follows:

High	greater than 135
Medium	between 120 and 135 (inclusive)
Low	below 120.

Then IQ can be treated as a factor with three levels. Similar treatment for Attitudes and Practice could be carried out, and the data could then be analysed through ANOVA. However, note that by treating each of the variables in this way, some of the information in the data is being lost – no distinction is made between IQs of 121 and 131, for example. This loss of information inevitably results in a reduction in statistical *power*. A further point is that basic ANOVA treats Low, Medium, High as simply three different levels, and takes no account of the fact that the levels are ordered. However, that is not a particular problem – to take account of this ordering, follow-up trend tests would be appropriate (see page 203).

ANOVA and MRA may be contrasted in many ways:

■ While they are related mathematically, the basic way of talking about ANOVA analyses is in terms of comparing means (relative to variation), while the basic way of talking about MRA analyses is in terms of correlations. These contrasts reflect the way in which ANOVA may be considered as a generalisation of t-tests and MRA a generalisation of correlation and regression with a single predictor variable.

■ There are differences in terminology. Thus, the independent variables for ANOVA are called factors, while for MRA the independent variables are called predictor variables, and the dependent variable is called the criterion variable.

■ ANOVA is best suited for manipulated variables, that is, variables under the control of the experimenter and taking a small number of values. Variables such as IQ have to be banded artificially into a small number of intervals (for example, high, medium, low) if they are to be included as factors in an ANOVA design. MRA, on the other hand, is naturally suited to variables such as IQ that come with the participants, so to speak.

■ Related to the previous point, ANOVA is more suited to controlled laboratory research, whereas MRA is suited to research outside the laboratory, where there is less chance of experimental control.

■ An ANOVA design imposes restraints, particularly in the ideal case where the numbers of participants in all cells of a factorial design are equal. The reward for this discipline is that the interpretation of the results is straightforward. ANOVA divides the variation in the data into neat, discrete, packets – so much for each main effect, so much for each interaction, and so much background variation. By contrast, MRA is much more flexible, but the price paid for this flexibility is that interpretation often is not straightforward, particularly when predictors are themselves highly correlated.

CHAPTER REVIEW

In this chapter, you have been introduced to the techniques of multiple regression analysis, with a range of examples showing its flexibility. The basic building block underlying the logical structure of these examples is the regression model for the relationship between a set of predictor variables and a criterion variable, and comparisons between such models. A survey of the many contrasts between ANOVA and MRA concluded the chapter.

Overview

**IN THIS CHAPTER
. . .**

. . . we review the key ideas of the book and show how these fit within the cyclical process of experimentation and theory-building in psychology. We discuss the centrality of significance testing in traditional approaches to statistical inference in psychological research, the controversies relating to this approach, and various ways to supplement it, indicating the directions in which your statistical knowledge will need to be extended if you want to take your statistical education further. We finish with some reflections on the nature and aims of the book as a whole.

ON SEEING THE WOOD FOR THE TREES: WHAT ARE THE BIG IDEAS?

VARIABILITY

If we had to nominate one idea as the most important in understanding statistical analysis of data from psychological research, it would be variability. In a nutshell, as discussed in Chapter 1, variability is characteristic of the subject matter of psychology, namely people. Statistical methods are the techniques devised to cope with this most human of characteristics in attempting to understand people through empirical enquiry, and establish data-based theoretical generalisations about them.

VARIABLES

To be able to handle variability, both conceptually and mathematically, the building block is the concept of a variable, by which is meant, broadly speaking, any aspect within the experimental situation that varies and can be measured on a single scale.

Subject variables are characteristics of the people being studied (for example, gender, age, IQ, level of anxiety). Whereas a variable such as age or gender may be considered reasonably straightforward to define, examples of variables such as IQ and anxiety are complex and themselves embedded in theory – for example, it is highly controversial whether it is appropriate or not to measure intelligence on a single scale. As discussed in Chapter 2, a major effort of psychologists is in postulating and defining viable and useful variables and then devising, often with considerable ingenuity, ways of measuring them.

Treatment variables are aspects of the experimental conditions under the control of the experimenter, depending on the nature of the experiment – such as the nature of reinforcement, whether the participant is given coffee or not, and so on.

Both subject and treatment variables give rise to numbers, which may be as simple as 0 and 1 representing a dichotomous variable, such as gender or having/not having coffee. These numbers, organised variable by variable, are the raw materials for statistical analysis.

PROCESS OF EXPERIMENTATION

As has already been seen in Chapters 1 and 9, the process of experimentation broadly follows the stages shown in Figure 15.1.

■ A round in the ongoing cyclical process of experimentation and theory-building begins with the posing of a question in the form of a conjectured relationship among two or more variables (the experimental hypothesis).

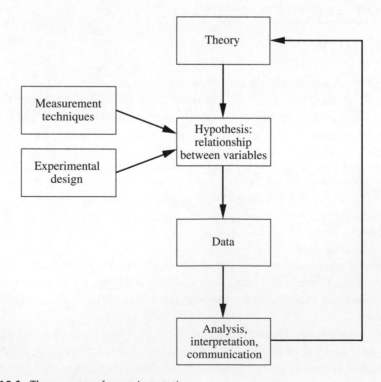

Figure 15.1 The process of experimentation

- In order to be able to investigate this conjectured relationship statistically, it must be possible to measure each variable.

- An experimental design is needed so that the data that the experiment generates appropriately bear on the theoretical question of interest.

- The data collected are analysed, interpreted, and communicated. The interpretation feeds back into theory development.

INFERENCE FROM SAMPLE TO POPULATION

Given that the aim of building theory is to make statements about people in general, and given that it is obviously impossible to study everyone, psychological researchers have no option but to collect data for only a sample of the people of interest (say 12-year-old children, or left-handed people).

As a natural consequence of variability, a sample may not be representative of the population from which it is drawn – if a different sample is taken, the results may be very different. Think of a bag with fifty red marbles and fifty green marbles in it. Pull out ten marbles at random. They might all be red, they could all be green, or anything in between. If we do it many times, the number of red and green marbles will fluctuate markedly from one time to the next.

Now think of a bag with 100 marbles, each of which is red or green. Somebody picks out ten at random, of which six are red and four are green. What are the possibilities? All you know for certain is that six are red and four are green. The number of red marbles originally in the bag could be anything from six to ninety-six.

Trying to analyse data from a psychological experiment is like seeing the six red and four green marbles and *never being allowed to see inside the bag*. So how can we ever find out about what is in the bag? This is where the part of mathematics called the theory of probability comes to our aid (see Chapter 6). While it is true that randomly taking ten marbles from a bag with fifty red and fifty green could result in the number of reds being anything from none to ten, the theory of probability tells us that it is highly unlikely that it will be as extreme as zero or ten. To be more specific, it tells us that the probability is greater that 95 per cent that the number of reds will lie between two and eight (inclusive). Similarly, for the bag for which we don't know how many marbles are red and how many green, drawing out six red and four green allows us to *estimate* that there are sixty red and forty green marbles in the bag, and further analysis can quantify the likely ranges for the number of red and green marbles (say with a probability of 95 per cent).

In short, an intuitive acceptance of sampling variation is one of the key insights in truly understanding the principles of statistical analysis. A second, related, key insight is that, to put in the most general terms, probabilistic phenomena stabilise as the number of cases becomes very large.

By way of example, think of tossing a (fair) coin ten times. The probability that the number of heads will lie between four and six is .66 (to two decimal places). Now think in terms of proportions. In these terms, the probability that the number of heads will lie between 40 per cent and 60 per cent is .66. Now suppose the coin is tossed 100 times. The probability that the percentage of heads lies between 40 per cent and 60 per cent is now greater than .95. Increase the number of coin tosses to 1000 and the probability of the percentage of heads lying between 40 per cent and 60 per cent is extremely close to 1. In fact, there is a probability of about .95 that the percentage of heads in this case (for 1000 coin tosses) lies between 47 per cent and 53 per cent.

This pervasive characteristic of probabilistic phenomena (exemplified at many points throughout this book) explains why the number of participants tested in a given experiment is a vital factor in determining the power of the statistical test carried out (see Chapter 9).

EVALUATING THE VALUE OF A STATISTIC

The term *statistical inference* refers to the necessity of making an inference about a population on the basis of data collected for a sample of that population. Such an inference from sample to population is made through a statistic, which is a number derived from the data that expresses a specific and relevant aspect of the data. Throughout the book, in introducing each statistic, we have emphasised the logic of its definition in terms of what aspect of the data it measures. For example, the Mann–Whitney U statistic (see page 110) reflects the degree to which data from the two groups being compared are mixed up or not when they are combined and listed in order. The independent t-test (see page 103) is the ratio of the difference between means for scores from two independent groups to a measure of the variation in these scores within these groups that also takes sample size into account; examples were presented in Chapter 7 to explain the rationale for this definition of the statistic.

In general (all things being equal) the strength of the evidence that the data provide in terms of evaluating the experimental hypothesis is related directly to the size of the statistic, as we have emphasised throughout, in particular through the use of schematic diagrams (see, for example, Figure 7.13). For an independent groups design for example, the t statistic can potentially take any value, positive or negative. All else being equal, the further away from zero (whether positive or negative), the stronger the evidence of a difference in the population in the characteristic under study. As repeatedly stressed, the question then is: just how far away from zero does the t value have to be before we consider it as constituting strong enough evidence of a difference?

A similar question arises for each statistic we have dealt with, and we have described in this book the most generally used method in psychological statistics for answering this question, based on the concept of the null hypothesis and examining the implications of assuming it to be true. In fact, such is the ubiquity of the approach, many textbooks present it as the sole method for evaluating data. The null hypothesis method yields a way of deciding what range of values of a statistic are deemed to satisfy the very specific criterion that is termed *statistical significance*. While the approach continues to be dominant, there are major controversies surrounding it, to which we now turn.

LIMITATIONS OF THE NULL HYPOTHESIS APPROACH

The approach we have described for determining whether a statistic is, or is not, statistically significant has been standard for a long time in psychological research. However, essentially for as long as it has been used, it has also been criticised on many counts. Furthermore, whereas, in the past, much publication of statistical experiments concentrated on reporting whether the results of tests were statistically significant or not, there is now considerable pressure to provide further information. If you are going to take your statistics education further, you will need to go deeper into such matters; here we sketch briefly the main forms of criticism, and some suggested ways to meet them.

You may be surprised, and perhaps somewhat dismayed, to be told that what you have painstakingly (we hope) been learning is based on controversial foundations. However, even the physical sciences are built on an edifice that is no longer seen as incontrovertibly true, but rather a set of theories of models that we construct in an attempt to explain the physical world – think of the arguments surrounding Darwinian theories of evolution, for example. Because statistical methods draw on the mathematical theory of probability, it might be imagined that they thereby acquire the certainty of mathematics, but the theoretical foundations of probability are themselves uncertain. In every respect, we live in an uncertain world, and absolute certainty is not even to be found in mathematics.

At the root of the criticism of the statistical approach based on evaluating the null hypothesis is being clear about what 'statistical significance' actually tells us. In Chapter 6, we tried to make this point as clearly as possible. In particular, the statement that a result is *statistically significant at the .05 level* is a statement about the probability of getting a value of the statistic in a certain range, on the assumption that the null hypothesis is true. It is, emphatically, *not a statement about the probability of the null hypothesis being true*. The all-too-easy tendency to slide between the correct interpretation and the incorrect one is an example of confusing conditional probabilities, as explained in Chapter 6. Research has shown that the error is pervasive, even among experienced researchers, and is propagated in many textbooks (not this one, is our earnest hope).

Thus, what the statistical significance of a result tells you is rather limited, and in a sense 'indirect'. It may be regarded as a minimal safeguard against reading incorrectly into data evidence for a systematic effect that is not warranted. If you continue with your statistical education, you will need to extend beyond mere determination of whether a result is statistically significant or not, and consider other aspects of the data.

In particular, in this book, we have touched only very lightly on the importance of the power of an experiment, yet it is well known that in psychological research many experiments are based on sample sizes which imply that their power is undesirably low. This reality has a cumulatively distorting effect on how experimental data feed back into theory-building, since it implies that many experiments fail to yield statistically significant results that would have been produced by larger samples (or more carefully designed experiments). For your future statistical education, you will need to know a lot more about power and how it can be calculated for specific experimental designs.

Another aspect is that the use of the word 'significance' is unfortunate in that it carries the message that a statistically significant result is significant in the general sense of the word, which is not necessarily the case. Because of the ever present effect of sample size, a statistically significant effect can be obtained with a very large sample which represents a very small difference between two means, for example, or a very small correlation. Indeed, a correlation of .01, or even lower, is statistically significant if the sample size is large enough.

As we saw in Chapter 9 (page 165), the magnitude of the Pearson correlation coefficient (r) is itself a measure of **effect size** – the strength of the systematic relationsip in the data that is independent of statistical significance. For experimental designs such as an independent groups design, the effect size can also be given as a value between 0 and 1 and, unlike a t value, which is dependent on N, it takes account of the sample size in its calculation, so that experiments with different numbers of perticipants can be directly compared. Similar calculations can be carried for ANOVA and chi-square designs. Effect size is an aspect of data analysis that is increasingly coming into prominence as earlier concentration on reporting statistical significance alone is perceived to be inadequate.

Another way in which more valuable information can be presented is in the form of **confidence intervals**. You may well have seen reports of opinion polls or electoral polls in which, let's say for the sake of example, it is reported that 31 per cent of those polled considered that cats are better companions than dogs, and this is followed by the statement 'margin of error ±3%'. You will certainly realise that this does not mean that the actual percentage of the population who think that cats are better companions than dogs lies in the range from 28 per cent to 34 per cent. What it means is that, roughly speaking (and an exact explanation of what we mean here by 'roughly speaking' is beyond the scope of this book), there is a 95 per cent probability that the percentage lies in that range. The advantage of this extra information is that it not only gives us an estimate of the pro-cat percentage in the population, but also an indication of the precision of that estimate. As another example of the importance of sample size, the margin of error in a case like this is directly related to the size of the poll – interview fewer people and the margin of error increases; interview more and it decreases.

In a similar way, confidence intervals can be calculated for statistics. For example, if a correlation coefficient of .42 is reported, it can be augmented by a statement that the 95 per cent confidence interval is, say, .36 to .48 (the actual value will depend on the sample size, of course), which again means (roughly) that there is a 95 per cent probability that the true value lies in that range.

What the foregoing paragraphs represent, then, are sketchy indications of the ways in which the null hypothesis approach to statistical inference is deemed to be controversial, and of ways in which the reporting of statistical significance can be augmented by other information necessary to evaluate the significance, in the general sense, of the data.

MAKING SENSE OF A MULTIVARIATE WORLD

The important questions about people are complex. More specifically, to understand complex aspects of behaviour, many variables need to be taken into account. In Part I of this book, we limited attention to simple experimental designs involving at most two variables – these are important enough in their own right, and serve to establish a foundation for moving on to the more powerful experimental designs dealt with in Part II.

In Chapters 10 to 13 on ANOVA, we showed how the analysis of data by comparing means relative to variation within groups could be extended, first by having more than two levels of the independent variable, and then by increasing the number of independent variables to two or more. Such designs allow the effects of several independent variables to be taken into account and, moreover, possible interactions between two or more to be considered, something not enabled by a series of simpler experiments, each with one independent variable. The case of interaction in ANOVA exemplifies the point that, in describing and understanding complex behaviour, intricate patterns within data for many variables need to be teased out. In a relatively simple example (see page 213) we saw that comparing males and females on recognition of specific sets of photographs could only be interpreted meaningfully by taking into account a third variable, namely the nature of the groups of people in the photographs (in this case, models, footballers, or pop stars).

In Chapter 14, regression analysis was extended in similar fashion to encompass data where multiple variables could be treated as predictors. The examples given to illustrate the flexibility of the approach show various ways in which it serves to tease out the relationships between several variables. For example, on page 245, when dealing with which factors influence attitudes to computers among psychology students, five potentially important predictors were considered, namely Faculty, Gender, IQ, External Locus of Control, and Computer use. On the basis of the data available for a reasonably large sample of students, it appeared that only External Locus of Control and Computer use were the important predictors out of the set considered. Again, if you are going to go further with statistics, one direction in which your skill and knowledge will be extended is in learning more multivariate methods designed to cope with our multivariate world.

Figure 15.2 completes the picture of the landscape sketched in this book. Taking account of the contents of Part II, the diagram is an elaboration of Figure 9.10.

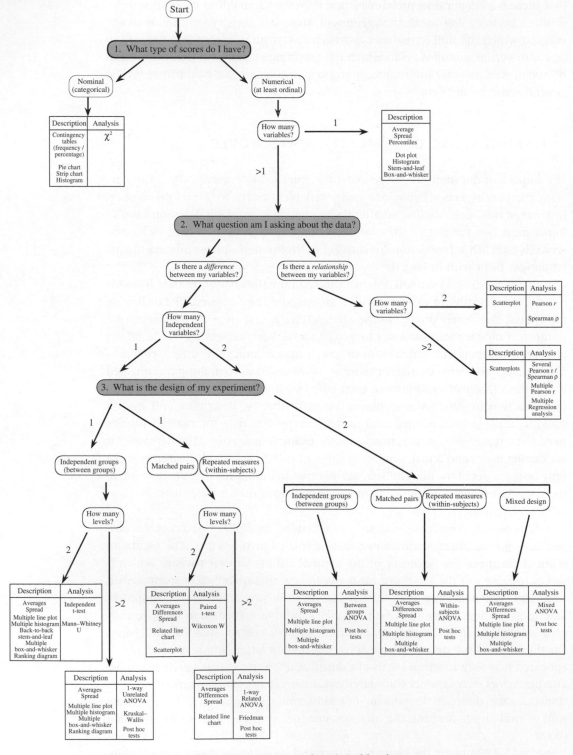

Figure 15.2 Decision chart: overview of statistical landscape

In selecting a statistical approach to any data set, you may find it useful to refer to this diagram, or Figure 9.10, for less advanced tests. Again for ease of access, Figure 15.2 is reprinted on the *back inside cover*. Regular reference to these figures will help you to acquire a reliable schema for statistics. You may be interested to note that, in spite of the inclusion of more statistical techniques in Figure 15.2, the relationship between tests continues to be governed by the same three basic questions introduced in Chapter 9.

BOOK REVIEW

In some senses, our ambitions in this book have intentionally been limited. In spite of our foregoing comments on the directions in which your future statistical education is likely to go, in terms of content we have largely restricted ourselves to, as it were, the orthodoxy in undergraduate psychological statistics. We have tried to balance a desire to break certain moulds, and to look towards future trends, with a realistic sense of what students and teachers of statistics believe they need *now – today*. Mindful of these not entirely compatible concerns, we have attempted to house introductory statistics and research methods, as well as a solid conceptual foundation in post-introductory statistics, under the same roof.

Again, intentionally, there are many details of both elementary and post-elementary statistics that we have omitted – in trying to help you see the wood for the trees, we have cleared away quite a lot of the undergrowth. We don't imagine that you have been cast up alone on a desert island with this book – we expect you to supplement it by additional reading and by benefiting from your statistics instruction. Thus, while we have endeavoured to cover the main points in a coherent way we have, above all, attempted to provide a solid conceptual framework.

Statisticians and mathematicians might be shocked at the lack of formulae and technical derivations throughout the book – on this point we are unrepentant. We have taken for granted that you have access to powerful statistical software, without tieing our discussion (as many texts do) to a particular package. There is simply no point, in our opinion, in presenting complex formulae to students, when most of them lack the technical facility to understand the mathematics. In our experience, many introductory texts claim to eschew mathematical complexity in favour of conceptual explanations, but this aim rarely lasts beyond about Chapter 3; we trust we have done better in this respect.

In a deeper sense, however, we have been extremely ambitious. We have attempted, based on our long experience of teaching a population of psychology undergraduates, to present a book that you will find interesting and accessible, and will provide a conceptual framework for, as the title implies, making sense of data and statistics in psychology, whether this is the last statistics you study formally, or whether you go on to become a researcher or a statistical expert.

If you intend to become a researcher, the case for understanding statistics hardly needs to be made. If not, there is still a very high chance that your work will involve dealing with complex issues involving people. Statistical tools for interpreting and communicating data will almost certainly be important in any such career.

Beyond pragmatic considerations of your future career, it is clear that basic statistical literacy is essential in our contemporary world, where there is a proliferation of data, mostly presented by agencies such as governments, pressure groups, the media, or advertisers, that have a vested interest in persuasion. In this environment, a critical disposition allied with a feel for data and an expectation that it should be possible to make sense of data for yourself, are vital. Given the Internet and other aspects of the information explosion, the ratio

$$\frac{\text{Amount of available information}}{\text{Conceptual tools for making sense of it}}$$

is liable to increase out of control. We hope this book helps.

Index